D1443376

WHEN WOMEN RISE

WHEN WOMEN RISE

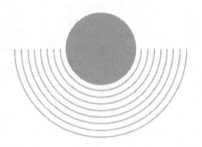

Everyday Practices to Strengthen
Your Mind, Body, and Soul

DR. MICHELE KAMBOLIS

Figure.1
Vancouver / Berkeley

Cataloguing data is available from Library and Archives Canada
ISBN 978-1-77327-156-9 (hbk.)
ISBN 978-1-77327-157-6 (ebook)
ISBN 978-1-77327-158-3 (pdf)

Design by Naomi MacDougall
Author photograph by Candace Meyer
Editing by Lesley Cameron
Copy editing by Lucy Kenward
Proofreading by Marnie Lamb
Indexing by Marnie Lamb

Printed and bound in Canada by Friesens
Distributed internationally by Publishers Group West

Figure 1 Publishing Inc.
Vancouver BC Canada
www.figure1publishing.com

This book is dedicated to my grandmother
Eunice, who truly radiates unconditional love.

And to the many women who have so
courageously shared their life stories with me.
Without their heart wisdom this book would
never have happened.

CONTENTS

MEDITATIONS

BREATHING EXERCISES

MANTRA

RELAXATIONS

Introduction

OVER THE PAST twenty-two years I've worked with thousands of women. So many of them have said the same thing: "Something just isn't working in my life." They've wanted to feel happier and more complete, suffer less, and live in a more expansive and empowered way. Perhaps most of all, they've wanted to heal their heart and mind and nurture their sacred connection to life, but the options to do so are frequently out of reach. Not many of us have the financial means or the time to attend the workshops and expensive trainings that make up the modern wellness industry. That's why I've written *When Women Rise*. It honors every woman's right to access scientifically supported practices to reawaken and reconnect with her already perfect self.

In this book we'll look honestly at every aspect of ourselves—mind, body, and soul. We'll open new dimensions of possibility and discover a deep inner knowing that lives beyond the self-limiting stories being replayed in our minds and the cultural pressures we face every day. Restoring and maintaining our well-being comprises three primary tasks. To master our mind, we must learn to be mindful and compassionately aware. To master our body, we must learn to both honor our body and strengthen it with nature's medicine. To master our spiritual lives, we must tend to the sacred within. Working on these three tasks will help us not only undo the deep conditioning that holds us back from reaching our highest well-being but also learn to love and be at home with ourselves.

We'll move through these tasks with a broad range of systematic tools and practices that can transform your perspective and change your habits. Some practices may seem like common sense and others may seem more mysterious. All draw on the science of mind-body medicine and, crucially, have been tested in real-life situations by the thousands of women I've had the good fortune to work with. They will help you tend to the physical, emotional, and spiritual aspects of your life as one inextricably intertwined unit. How each of us defines spirit may be deeply personal. But whether you see it as nature, a vitality within and around you, a life force, a higher intelligence, or consciousness beyond the physical form, these practices will nurture and honor it.

In the pages of this book you'll find scientifically supported ways to stimulate healing by listening to the subtle cues of your mind-body system, signs of imbalance so often overlooked or ignored. You'll build your capacity for enduring health with a framework that moves well past the Western model. With a more open, layered, and holistic approach to healing, you'll have access to a centuries-old wisdom that's as valid today as it was when it was first developed.

I'll guide you through a discovery of your inner patterns, daily habits, and choices that support or hinder your sense of fulfillment. You'll become a little more conscious of where you're slipping into patterns of behavior that no longer serve you. Every woman's process of discovery will be different. What you choose to integrate into your life will be unique to you. You may find yourself going through the doorways of breath work, or perhaps meditation or the alchemy of sleep will speak most intimately to you. Whichever portals you step through, you will find yourself at the same destination: yourself.

The practices don't require you to devote hours of your day to them, but you do need to give them a chance. A single meditation probably won't change your life. With regular practice, however, you'll find they have the potential to rewire your mind and body in profoundly transformative ways. You'll find yourself creating new patterns based in greater awareness, compassion, and equanimity and naturally creating a life that is guided by wisdom and an intuitive sense of what serves your greatest aspirations. What you practice, you will embody.

Whenever I start a meditation class or a therapeutic session with a client, we take a moment together to root firmly in the purpose and intention of our healing work. When an intention is rooted in clarity, and positive emotions like joy and enthusiasm, life can transform in miraculous ways. That intention becomes our reference point as we weave and design the practices that heal, strengthen, and transform. We draw on our innate courage and wisdom and allow intention and life to become one. We do this work not only for ourselves but also for the healing and peace of all.

I invite you to set your own intention now. Each time you return to the practices in this book, remind yourself of the deepest wishes you hold for yourself. Perhaps you want to feel calmer, more joyful, empowered, or connected. Or perhaps you have big and exciting dreams and you'd like to remove the internal obstacles that are preventing you from achieving them. Aspirations are like signposts: they guide us along life's journey and allow us to reflect on where we are.

Although each chapter can stand alone as a source of information, all the chapters are interrelated and knowing more about one topic will enhance your learning experience of another. For that reason, I encourage you to start at the beginning of the book, work your way to the end, and return to whichever chapters speak most to you. In particular, if you're new to meditation, you might want to carefully read the section below on cultivating your meditation practice to get comfortable with the process. Rereading chapters or your journal entries, or notes you have made in the margins of these pages, can help you integrate new knowledge, health habits, and personal reflections. And earlier chapters may take on new meaning as you change and grow, or a significant life event may call you back to a certain part of the book. Think of this process as an invitation to let go of the Western pattern of pushing, forcing, and chasing and begin to challenge the unexamined patterns that interfere with your ability to be fully present to the richness of your life as it is right here, right now. Let's begin.

Cultivating a Meditation Practice

Meditation is a golden ticket to making peace with ourselves. It has endless mind-body health benefits and is foundational to many of the practices in this book. All forms of meditation strengthen the conditions essential to enduring happiness and well-being, but it can be hard for new meditators to make it to their mats every day. Our lives are so caught up in the "doing" that "non-doing" just doesn't seem so feasible.

Hands down the biggest barrier to starting a regular practice is our own resistance to coming face-to-face with our mind. We doubt ourselves, worry that we somehow can't meditate, tell ourselves that we just don't have the time. I can honestly say, as long as you're breathing, you do have enough time, you can sit still, and meditation isn't just for yogis. As part of my doctoral research, I've had some fascinating discussions with people who have meditated daily for over thirty or forty years about how their practice informs their lives. I've learned they have a whole host of habits that support them in developing a meditation practice that they've maintained. For example, setting an attitude of openness can make all the difference. You might start your practice by placing the hand at the heart and saying to yourself, "May I keep an open heart and mind, so I may give myself fully to this moment."

For most meditators, formal practice is easier in the morning, when information from the day has yet to be downloaded. Sitting every day, even if it's for a short period, will help build those meditation muscles. Some people meditate for a short time two or three times per day; others sit once for a longer period. It can be helpful to choose a specific length of time for your practice and gradually increase it each day. For many beginning meditators, five to ten minutes is a good place to start.

Your relationship with meditation is deeply personal and yours to develop according to what works best for you. If you miss a day or two, or twenty, don't worry. Simply begin again. Your practice isn't punitive and it welcomes you back at each return.

Invitations to Practice

Throughout these pages are many exercises that invite you to practice. They are entry points for healing, exploring, and embarking on a wondrous journey of inner knowing. You may try the exercises once or return to them again and again. They will help you to integrate new knowledge, and I encourage you to practice them in the order they're shown while the learning is fresh in your mind. You'll find eighteen meditations as well as imagery exercises, breathing techniques, mantras, biofeedback strategies, mindfulness practices, and an entire system predicated on mind-body health and self-knowing. These evidence-based practices are an all-encompassing guide deeply rooted in neuroscience, psychology, and integrative medicine. Some exercises have their own QR code that leads to a recording.

Every moment dedicated to practice counts. Some exercises may feel unpleasant and others will feel so good you'll want to do them again and again. Value them equally and keep in mind that this practice isn't about achieving a certain state; it's about opening our eyes to what's there and experiencing ourselves fully.

This book is filled with questions designed to take you deeper into self-knowing. Instead of choosing only the questions that inspire you, make sure to sit with the ones you are resisting. Those often tell us more about ourselves than the ones that feel inviting and bring pleasure. The key is writing your responses down. Seeing your thoughts and feelings on paper can significantly expand your awareness, help you confront your assumptions, and motivate you toward a life that is aware, wise, and true to you.

This will be an active journey of transformation, and the journaling process will help inspire an inner shift when you need it the most. Use the journal prompts at the end of each chapter to help integrate the material and examine what it means in your life. Use them to help you keep track of new awarenesses and to guide you into deeper contemplation. And don't underestimate the value of rereading old entries. It can be fascinating to see the ways in which our perceptions and attitudes are changing.

The practices in this book will support you in accelerating the evolution of consciousness that is already taking place on this planet. Every woman has the capacity to break free from ingrained patterns and step into her greatest freedom, her true and authentic self. May this practice serve you well as you transcend your fears and reclaim the self-determination that is your birthright.

The Wisdom of the Buddha Within

When I was a teenager I stumbled across a book called *The Hermit* about a Tibetan *lama* (teacher), and something about the story left me so intrigued by the mystery of meditation that I began looking for ways to learn more. My first boyfriend had recently died in a violent car accident, and I took refuge in the quiet sanctuary of my community library. There, the book opened a pathway to learn how to be with the grief and regret, and the relentless thoughts of guilt, in ways that no longer sat so heavily in my heart. In time, meditation taught me ways to watch and notice and observe as the pain arose, existed, and dissolved. The practices I learned gave my sixteen-year-old self a life raft to help carry me through my almost unbearable loss. For decades to come I would fall in and out of practice, commit, fall asleep, and recommit. Eventually, meditation stopped becoming an item on my to-do list and became an intimate and integral part of my life.

Several years ago, I opened *The Hermit* again. I had carried it with me for over thirty-five years. I wanted to know more about the wise Tibetan lama who had soothed me in a time of intense grief and set me on a life-changing path. It turned out that the author wasn't a Tibetan lama at all. He was a plumber living in Alberta, Canada. I learned then that the wisdom of the Buddha really does lie within each of us, and our greatest teachers can come in unexpected forms.

Throughout the last two decades of my clinical practice, my clients have primarily been women, and in that time I have come to understand the barriers and struggles of women intimately. As someone who was born and identifies as female, I know all too well

the impacts of sexism, and the oppression, disempowerment, financial stress, sexual harassment, and many other struggles women face
because of gender inequality. I also understand what's possible when
we feel safe in our own bodies, empower and honor one another with
an eye to our innate strength, and have equal opportunity to develop
our potential to its fullest. *When Women Rise* is for anyone who
wishes to discover and address the physical, emotional, and spiritual
vitality of those who identify as women.

A LITTLE NOTE OF ENCOURAGEMENT

I often see women carrying a tremendous amount of
guilt as they take steps toward greater self-care. The
story they've been told is that self-care is indulgent
or selfish. In truth, self-care isn't selfish and it isn't
trivial—it's your birthright. Life is an ongoing practice
of self-care. When you drink a cup of herbal tea, sigh
a long exhale, hold a moment of appreciation, or walk
to the store rather than drive, you're honoring yourself
with self-care. So when you find yourself searching
to justify taking your full lunch break or feeling guilty
about asking the kids to play on their own because you
want to turn inward with a little journaling, try this
exercise instead.

Take a moment to close your eyes, be aware of yourself as light, and let that light travel all the way up to the
cosmos. Sit on a star. As your spirit rests, take a low
and slow breath in, and from this bird's-eye perspective
gaze down at yourself with compassionate awareness.
Notice just how hard your body is working to sustain
you faithfully. It asks very little and is extraordinarily forgiving. When you're ready, return to the body and in a
soft whisper let it know, "I thank you and I've got you."

The Welcoming

TIME NEEDED: 4 MINUTES

This meditation was inspired by the teachings of social justice activist Konda Mason, whose guidance has helped so many people examine with fresh eyes the dynamics of oppression and inclusion.

LET'S BEGIN BY coming into stillness.

You might close your eyes or leave them open slightly, resting the gaze lightly on the space in front of you.

There is no wrong way to be here.

Welcome yourself into this moment.

There is no better thing to do with time today than this.

Let this be a loving practice of self-discovery.

Notice the breath now, and the body.

Take in a deep sense of welcome.

Allow yourself to soften at the heart center.

And know that every part of you is welcomed here.

Together, let us welcome all genders.

We welcome all of the backgrounds and languages that you bring.

We welcome your diverse races and ethnic groups, all sexual orientations, and faiths.

We welcome your diverse bodies and abilities, and people of all ages.

We welcome those who are single, married, parents, nonparents. We welcome all of you.

We welcome all your emotions, your worries and fear, and your joy.

Let us welcome each other with the heart of unwavering love and respect.

And may we rise into our highest well-being together.

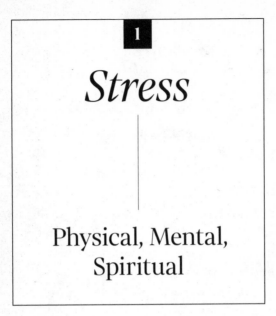

Stress

Physical, Mental, Spiritual

"*We are capable of so much more than we usually dare to imagine.*"

SHARON SALZBERG, author and cofounder of the Insight Meditation Society

Maya's Story

Maya smiled at me warmly, settling into the corner of the sofa. We'd met several times previously and I found myself sinking into a sense of intimacy, a familiarity of connection. "What are you noticing?" I asked her. It's an invitation to awareness, often met with a sigh of relief. She adjusted the wisps of her bangs with a nervousness I hadn't seen in her before.

"What am I noticing? Good question," she said. She sat, waited, scanned, and began again. "Tightness in my chest. My breath is shallow. Anxiety, racing thoughts. It's not a lot of fun in here. What

I'm feeling most is a sense of failure. And shame." She seemed more open than in other sessions, vulnerable. She continued, "I don't have a moment to just breathe. The kids are up by six and my husband says he'll look after them but doesn't. He hasn't made it home before eight in over a week because, of course, his career comes first, and I'm exhausted." I could easily have been talking to my younger self. And then her inner critic took over: "I don't know what's wrong with me. I've been on anti-anxiety medication for months. I try to meditate, eat well, exercise when I can, and still my mind won't stop." I'd seen her long enough to know that there was so much more to her story. Anyone who knows or spends time with Maya can easily see her perfectionism. What they couldn't see was her pain.

Maya's parents divorced when she was in grade school and she saw her father very little. Her brother had a full-ride basketball scholarship to university, while she struggled to pay for an arts degree. She'd had a mild eating disorder throughout her twenties and then married into a family highly focused on achieving wealth and status. She'd tried to conceive for two years before she had her two children. But the therapy notes don't capture the deeper under-current of Maya's struggles. After her parents separated, Maya's mother relied on her heavily for emotional support. When Maya most needed to be cared for, she became the caregiver instead. While her younger brother played with friends, she did chores. When her mother cried, Maya hugged her tight. By the time Maya became a teenager she'd felt so responsible for her mother's grief and shame and unrealized dreams that her true self was nowhere to be found. Maya's need for her mother's approval had become crippling: each comment about her clothes, her weight, or her choice in boyfriends was like a pinprick of unmet expectation. She'd begun to look for external validation and love—though no number of achievements, smaller dress sizes, higher earnings, or social media attention could bring her the lasting fulfillment she so badly wanted.

Stress Is a Feminist Issue

Maya's struggle wasn't unlike those of many other women I work with, women who want desperately to transcend wounds from the past, the stressors of our cultural ecosystem, and physical and emotional impacts of those stressors. Her life was dominated by nurturing and caregiving—roles imposed predominantly on women by our patriarchal society—and the imbalance was taking a terrible toll on her mind, body, and spirit. Women's fatigue and stress go far beyond the need for better self-care, alone time, or support to get through the mounting daily tasks. Extra kale and yoga classes aren't going to help women change the early conditioning that tells us how to fit into a society dominated by masculine values and ideals. And they certainly aren't going to address the harder fact that women and girls in every country on our planet face discrimination, violence, financial and work inequity, and extraordinary challenges due to gender inequality. That's why I say stress is a feminist issue.

When we look at the history of women, we have to ask, Why wouldn't we be struggling with an extraordinarily high level of anxiety, trauma, and stress-related health crises? Every woman inherits the effects of trauma inflicted on the women who have come before her. If not through epigenetics (a growing area of research supporting the idea that trauma is biologically passed down through generations) then through our shared consciousness.[1] Women are actively taught from an early age to walk home at night with a friend for protection. We park near well-lit doorways and clench our keys defensively between our fingers as we make our way to our cars. We hold on to our drinks in pubs and restaurants for fear of being drugged. And we blame ourselves for being too nice when we're sexually harassed by our boss. We have learned to navigate our lives in fear.

Women in Western society are facing alarming levels of stress and anxiety. The costs to our health, emotional freedom, relationships with our children and partners, and society as a whole are too often overlooked. And when chronic stress becomes severe anxiety, the personal and societal costs of loss of work, hospital visits, unemployment, and impact on relationships can be devastating.[2] According to the National Institute of Mental Health in the United States, up to 19 percent of adults in America—that's 60 million people, or more than the entire population of Canada—have severe levels of anxiety in any given year.[3] Envision for a moment a sea of 60 million people before you, all suffering from anxiety. Imagine dividing that sea of people into four equal sections. In each section, include mothers, fathers, uncles, aunts, grandparents of every race, socioeconomic status, gender, educational level, and sexual orientation. Now picture yourself having to choose which of the four groups will be granted treatment. Only one out of four people with clinical levels of anxiety will ever get the help they need. Now take away a quarter of the men and replace them with women. Women are one-and-a-half times more likely to be affected by anxiety: that's nearly one in four women.[4] The question is, Why? (And remember, this is only clinical levels of anxiety. Imagine the numbers if we included people who fall below that medical threshold but are suffering nonetheless.)

Most literature attributes differences in anxiety between the male and female sexes to biological factors, stressing that hormones and brain chemistry must play a role.[5] However, cultural factors and women's lived experience tell the bigger story. Let's look at some statistics:

- Globally, one in three women experiences physical or sexual violence in her lifetime.[6]

- Worldwide, women who experience intimate partner violence—also referred to as domestic abuse, family violence, and gender-based violence—are twice as likely to suffer from depression or substance use.[7]

- Approximately 650 million women globally were child brides, married before the age of eighteen. In the past decade, one out of five women was married when she was a child.[8]

- Women do less paid and more unpaid work than men worldwide, working 25 unpaid minutes more per day than men. That may not seem like a lot, but in a 37.5-hour workweek that adds up to four additional weeks of work per year.[9]

- The gender pay gap in 2018 was 22% worldwide, leaving women earning only 78% of what men are paid.[10]

- Fewer than one in four parliamentarians worldwide is a woman.[11]

- Workplace sexual harassment was reported by 40 to 50% of women in the European Union.[12]

- Over 2.7 billion women lack job security, fair pay, and the same career opportunities as men.[13]

To compete in a male-dominated world, we do double shift, trying to be all things to all people. Women tell me how exhausted they are as they scramble to keep up, often feeling as though they're falling short. Single women feel they've failed because they haven't partnered or had children; those who have feel torn between career and mothering. If you belong to an ethnic minority, have a disability, are nonbinary, LGBTQIA+, or living in poverty, there's an intersection of oppression.

The Black socialist Claudia Jones brought to light in the 1940s and '50s the triple oppression that exists between classism, sexism, and racism. In her book *Women, Race & Class*, published in 1981, Angela Davis wrote about Claudia Jones and noted that she and other earlier generations of Black thinkers articulated the ideas that would become central to the Black feminist movement in the 1970s. Davis's book was a brave and seminal work by one of the first scholars to open our eyes to the fact that to end oppression we must tackle all its forms at once.[14]

In Western society, women try to adapt, strengthen, and build resilience to cope, only to be pushed back into an inequitable cultural ecosystem that has us breathing fear. We are led to believe that maternal employment is damaging to children, though studies have disproven this idea. And we struggle to balance work and home life, navigate the emotional minefield of social media, and withstand the pressure to be beautiful, accomplished, and visible. In truth, many women tell me they crave a wiser, more balanced way. Society's win-at-all-costs culture of competition has hurt them dearly. Their stressed-out bodies are telling them no more, not one more day of this unsustainable pressure. They are no longer willing to be judged by the standards of healthism—which believes that those who work out regularly, stay slim, and eat right are more worthy—or to see it as the answer to the much bigger social and political problem of chronic stress and toxic patriarchy.

Imagine all these women coming together in an unwavering spirit of compassion and strength. Envision challenging the cultural story we're told about who women are supposed to be, and instead forging a path of radical authenticity, self-realization, and self-care. Although each of us has our own path, the cumulative impact is profound. When one heals, the cultural needle moves a little farther and eventually our collective consciousness changes for the better.

The Central Nervous System

Although it's tempting to jump right into the deliciousness of inner work—meditating and journaling our way back to our well-being— it's difficult to attend to our inner world when our physical body needs attention. Imagine trying to give full presence and attention to your inner experience when your nervous system is taxed and you haven't slept well in days, or you're hungry because you've skipped your last meal, or your heart is racing from an argument you just had with your boss. If our physical and safety needs are not tended to, it's difficult to be present enough to give our fullest attention to the work of inner knowing and self-actualization. That's why you'll find a whole lot of mind-body health science running throughout this book. If you're not a science type, don't panic. The idea is to spark your curiosity about what's happening in that mysterious mind-body system of yours, so you're better equipped to respond when things are running less than smoothly. To know the body well is to see and hold in ourselves a care manual to create the kind of environment that supports us to be fully awake to our lives.

At the root of our well-being is our nervous system, the complex communication system of cells and nerves that carries messages to and from our brain, sensory organs, spinal cord, and various parts of our body. In its simplest definition, it is the system that determines and organizes our responses. Our nervous system coordinates voluntary movements (like the muscles that move our mouth when we speak) and involuntary movements (like the muscles that keep us breathing even while we're asleep). The system that controls our involuntary responses is called the autonomic nervous system and it can be divided into two parts: the sympathetic nervous system and the parasympathetic nervous system.

The sympathetic nervous system activates the fight-or-flight response during a threat or perceived danger and the parasympathetic nervous system restores the body to a state of calm. For example, the sympathetic nervous system causes us to sweat under stress or excessive heat, whereas the parasympathetic nervous system decreases our respiration and heart rate and puts us into a state of "rest and repair." I refer to these two aspects of the autonomic nervous system throughout the book, as well as a key component of the parasympathetic nervous system, the vagus nerve.

You'll also hear about the limbic system, which plays a key role in our health and well-being. It's the area of the brain that comprises a number of structures, including the amygdala and hippocampus, that communicate with the autonomic nervous system (through the pituitary gland). The limbic system interprets emotional responses, stores memories, and regulates hormones.

THE VAGUS NERVE

From the moment of our first breath we are set on a quest to feel safe in our bodies. The inner surveillance system monitoring whether we're in danger or not (known as neuroception) lies far beneath our conscious control. The vagus nerve plays the main role, responding to cues of safety and danger. It originates in the brain stem and extends down through the tongue, pharynx, vocal cords, organs, and gut. It communicates with our glands, influencing the production of anti-stress hormones and enzymes, which makes it a critical part of managing the stress response. It's like a cabling system integrating mind and body, its pathways serving as a communication system for the mind, heart, and gut instincts. The vagus is divided into the ventral (front) vagal pathway and the dorsal (back) pathway. A daily practice of tending to the vagus nerve gives an extraordinary payoff in that it helps to minimize feelings of anxiety and stress and return us to equilibrium. Later you'll learn the roles that breath work, meditation, mantras, and nutrition play in its overall health, but here's a potent tool to get you started.

Invitation to Practice: Vooo Chanting

Leading trauma therapist Peter Levine teaches a technique that helps to interrupt the mental and physical impact of stressful events.[15] I've found it to be highly effective for discharging the effects of trauma. It brings comfort in the midst of anxiety. It's called the Vooo technique (aptly named for the sound it makes) and involves directing the sound vibration to the gut as you exhale. The resonant sound stimulates the vagus nerve and shifts you out of the sympathetic nervous system's fight-or-flight response, which shuts down nonessential body systems, and into the parasympathetic nervous system's rest-and-repair response, which calms the body down. We also know that the vagus nerve stimulation resulting from Vooo chanting triggers a release of the neurotransmitter acetylcholine, which reduces heart rate and blood pressure, and supports digestion.

1. Find a comfortable place to practice. You might find it soothing to place one hand at the heart and the other at the belly. Settle into the body.

2. Take a deep, full breath, exhale, and make a sustained "vooo" sound as the air releases.

3. Make the tone nice and low and send the vibration directly to the gut.

4. Allow the next breath to find you, filling up the belly and chest, and begin again. Continue to "vooo" your way through the feelings of stress for as long as you need.

The Neurochemical System

Our human body is beautifully designed, equipped with everything we need to heal, grow, and thrive. Rich with hundreds of neurochemicals, our physiology nourishes us with pleasure and alerts us to pain. When we get to know them well, neurochemicals offer a gateway into what motivates our highs and lows and returns us to an inner balance. Beneath the surface, each neurochemical orchestrates a complex interplay of shifts in attention, mood, motivation, reactions, perception, sensation, and all kinds of other responses in the mind-body system. Now here comes the exciting part: our neurochemical system isn't a one-way process. We have the ability to influence and support this system in ways that leave us feeling calmer, and more connected and joyful. Although there are hundreds of neurochemicals in the body, let's meet some of our more influential ones, starting with those that make us feel good.

- **Dopamine:** This is the "pleasure neurochemical" associated with motivation and reward and the positive feelings that come with accomplishing a task. It plays a crucial role in our ability to think and plan for the future. It's the neurochemical that helps us to strive for things, and to find life interesting. It also causes arousal and can be released by kissing (as if we needed more reasons to kiss).

- **Endorphins:** The "calming neurochemicals" can be released through exercise and reduce our perception of pain. They can also be released through breath work when we align our breath to our heart rate. Endorphins are known as natural painkillers that can reduce stress and boost mood.

- **Gamma-aminobutyric acid (GABA):** This naturally occurring amino acid is a "calming" neurotransmitter that blocks impulses between nerve cells in the brain. By reducing these signals, it can decrease activity in the nervous system and help control fear and anxiety, which can have a relaxing effect. In fact, GABA supplements are a major component of many over-the-counter sleep medications.[16]

- **Oxytocin:** The "cuddle neurochemical" permeates our body, leaving us happier and less stressed. Especially important for attachment, it triggers the bond between a mother and her infant.[17] It's sometimes referred to as the "love drug" and plays an important role in fostering empathy, trust, sexual attraction, and relationship building. When oxytocin is released, our blood pressure and heart rate will lower, stress chemicals will plummet, and so too will pain (both emotional and physical).

- **Serotonin:** This is the "happiness neurochemical" that affects not only mood but every part of our body. It influences sleeping, eating, motor skills, and the healing of physical wounds. While it's often prescribed as an antidepressant medication in the form of a serotonin reuptake inhibitor (SSRI), it's a naturally occurring neurochemical that is primarily produced in the gut.

Now let's move over to the stress hormones.

- **Adrenaline (also known as epinephrine):** The "survival" hormone normally produced by the adrenal glands courses through our bloodstream in response to stress (known as the "adrenaline rush"). Our senses become more alert as our airways open up, increasing the supply of oxygen to the brain. Blood sugar (glycogen) and fats are released from the body's stores to provide quick energy, and pain is suppressed, which is why we can continue to run from a threat even if injured.[18]

- **Cortisol:** The "fight-or-flight" hormone produced by the adrenal glands courses through our bloodstream in response to stress. Elevated levels of cortisol wreak havoc on our mind-body health. This hormone amplifies anxiety, blood pressure, blood sugar levels, and pain sensitivity while suppressing immune function and the reproductive and digestive systems.[19]

While both adrenaline and cortisol are essential to our survival—adrenaline helps to regulate our metabolism and cortisol helps us to adapt to stress—problems arise when they are in oversupply or when they are released without a threat being present. The extra energy has no use and can result in restlessness, irritability, anxiety, and weight gain or loss.

Is All Stress Bad?

One of the most frequent questions I'm asked is this: Is all stress bad? It's a great question. After all, stress has affected every part of the natural world, shaping how we've developed and transformed as a species over the course of 4 million years. What would the outcome have been had we not become bipeds, two-footed beings with hands free to fend off predators and use tools?

Stress itself is not the enemy of our well-being. In fact, humans have not only endured stress but become better for it. Short-term, manageable stress primes our mind-body system to adapt, to think on our feet, and to perform at our best. Eustress (healthy stress) can bring us into a sense of flow and radiance so potent that it can feel somehow transcendental. It motivates us to reach toward the limit of our abilities and leads us into peak states. Eustress can be physically taxing to our body in the short term, but that stress fuels our resiliency, bolstering our immune system and our body's ability to recover. The stress response is our body's innate means to ensure our survival in the face of danger (real danger, that is). Short-term stress calls on the body's adrenaline response, also known as the fight-or-flight response, which primes the mind-body system to respond like a valiant and faithful warrior. This encoded wisdom has helped our species survive tribal warfare and attacks by saber-toothed tigers. The problem is that too many of us are now fighting phantom saber-toothed tigers.

The paradox is that over time the systems designed to help us thrive are pushing our nervous systems from stress to distress. A short-term, high-stakes work project becomes a long-term assignment; an acute health issue flares into a chronic condition; or an episodic disagreement with our partner erupts into an ongoing daily argument—you can see how easily the internal guidance systems can become taxed. The short-term stress that can be protective[20] and bolster our immune system becomes long-term stress that wears down our health on every level.

Chronic overexposure to cortisol and other stress hormones can disrupt almost all the body's processes, putting us at increased risk of a whole host of health problems.[21] It's been said that 75 percent of visits to a doctor's office are due to stress-related illnesses or conditions, such as digestive disorders, chronic pain, metabolic disorders, and heart disease. Yet, we continue to push through, working at the same pace and wondering why everyone else seems to be managing just fine under the same stressful conditions. The truth is that modern life is robbing us of our well-being. Addressing stress isn't a luxury—it's an outright necessity.

When Stress Becomes Anxiety

How can you tell when you've moved from adaptive stress to anxiety? Eliminate the stressor and see what happens. Take a week off work, for example, and just observe how you feel. If you can remove the stressor (easier said than done sometimes, I know), and the worry, panic, fatigue, anger, digestive problems, muscle tension, headaches, or difficulty focusing or remembering continue, then you may be living with the effects of anxiety. Anxiety exists when the symptoms persist but no external stressors are to be found.

When signals from the sympathetic nervous system alert us to perceived threat, the impact of stress is expressed physically through sweating, constant worrying, a pounding heart, and tense muscles (among other symptoms). The amygdala, the area of the brain that controls emotional processing, plays a pivotal role in the fight-or-flight response. This tiny almond-shaped section of the brain's nerve tissue filters incoming information and sends a warning about a perceived threat. Its nerve signals prompt the adrenal glands to

A LITTLE NOTE OF ENCOURAGEMENT

Although it may feel at first like you're carrying the meditation or breathing practice, eventually it will begin to carry you. Here are a few ways to help you settle into a structured practice. Decide on a schedule ahead of time, even if it's five minutes a day. State your intention out loud to those who can support you best to make yourself accountable. Ask a friend to join you so that you can be each other's accountability buddy. A structured practice will provide you with the learning space to both honor yourself and reshape your mind and body with life-changing habits. The more you practice, the more ease, flow, and automaticity you'll find in your day-to-day life. It's all well and good to find peace and clarity on the meditation mat or in your journal, but the test comes when your partner is irritable or you get cut off by another driver on the road. Life is the perfect teacher: every obstacle, every interaction, and every breath is an invitation to embodied practice.

release a surge of hormones, including adrenaline and cortisol. The body's stress response is usually self-limiting though. Once a perceived threat has passed, adrenaline and cortisol levels begin to drop, heart rate and blood pressure return to baseline levels, and other systems resume their regular activities. But when stressors are always present, that shutoff valve gets hijacked, leaving us feeling under attack, and the fight-or-flight reaction becomes relentlessly active.

The condition of chronic stress is as much psychospiritual as it is physical. We've faced crisis after crisis and lost the sacred natural rhythm that once was part of our lives. We find ourselves struggling to fit in practices that both enrich our inner world and protect us from the impact of stress. Instead, we default to more doing. And yet we know deep in our bones that there is a wiser way. We want to hold space for ourselves to be enlivened with well-being and we yearn to feel life more fully. We want to drop the habits that interfere with our ability to be the fullest expression of ourselves. And more than anything, we're tired of living in fear.

While not all of us have clinical levels of anxiety, none of us is immune to the experience of anxiety itself. And in my experience, most women do not recognize anxiety for what it is. The headaches, stomachaches, racing heart, insomnia, shortness of breath that go hand in hand with anxiety send women searching for answers from medical doctors and specialists. We go through test after test, and in time doctors rule out one diagnosis after another and exhaust all other possibilities. For many of us, this is the point at which we start on the path of deep inner work. This is the gift in anxiety: it's both an invitation into self-knowing and a master class in resiliency. It's the hard work that cracks our hearts open, builds our grit, and awakens us to a gentler, wiser way.

Anxiety forces us to sit up and take notice that we cannot continue to live this way. What we call the "anxious mind" in clinical practice is a mind that clouds our ability to see life as it truly is, stops us from doing that which we actually want to do, and stands between us and our goals and joys. It is filled with self-doubt and prevents us from trying something new, making the first move with someone we really like, or applying for a job that we've always wanted.

By learning about the impact of chronic stress and anxiety and the effect it has on the mind-body system, we become empowered with information. And by getting to know the nature of the mind-body intimately, we can begin to navigate our relationship with ourselves. And it is a relationship. In time, you'll communicate, solve problems, empathize, and soothe the mind-body much like you do with your partner, friend, or child. The message I want you to know—the one I wish I had been told myself—is that anxiety is not the enemy. It is our invitation to profound and meaningful growth.

If you've picked up this book, chances are you're looking to make some changes in your life. Maybe alarm bells in your body have been ringing loudly enough that you are sitting up and paying attention or you're uncomfortably aware that things could be better in one way or another. Anxiety whispers softly at first, but when left unaddressed it begins to bang at the door. All too often women suffer silently. In preparation for writing this book, I interviewed dozens of women about their struggles. They were facing fatigue, obsessive worry, a sense of powerlessness, fear, insomnia, headaches, irritability, and all kinds of other symptoms. Even though these conversations were happening during a time of pandemic, the patterns of suffering had begun much earlier in their lives.

Many of the symptoms of nervous system distress are internal, so they often go unnoticed by others for years, if not decades. Others can't see your racing thoughts, pounding heart, cold hands, exhaustion, or other symptoms. Most people with clinical levels of anxiety suffer for over ten years before they receive the right kind of help.[22] If this sounds like you, do not ignore your suffering or underestimate its effects and impact. While the practices in this book are deeply therapeutic and can help you heal from the effects of both milder and more extreme levels of anxiety, if you feel that anxiety is affecting your mental health, it might be time to reach out for conventional medical treatment. And if your concerns are unmet, reach out to someone else and keep reaching out until you're heard.

We all have our own unique personal struggles, and the impact of stress and anxiety may differ from one person to another. But common to all of us is the experience of suffering. In Buddhist terms, *dukkha* (suffering) is an innate characteristic we share. Your hurting heart makes you human. Difficulty is inherent to life and none of us is immune. Yet we blame ourselves or others for these unavoidable realities. Instead, we can look honestly at anxiety and other impacts of chronic stress and see it as an invitation to liberate ourselves from suffering. By paying attention to the unseen and unfelt parts of our psyche, we can recondition our relationship with ourselves and reconnect to a wholeness of being. This involves actively engaging in our own transformation and by extension the radical evolution of human consciousness itself.

The River of Awareness

TIME NEEDED: 10 MINUTES

THIS SIMPLE PRACTICE of arriving into receptive awareness is a wonderful entry point into the healing potential of meditation. It helps to decondition the stress reactions by witnessing the currents of thought as they arise, exist, and pass through the mind.

Settle into a comfortable position sitting cross-legged on the floor or perhaps on a chair.

Let the face be soft.

Relax at the shoulders.

Let the muscles release any tension collected there.

And allow yourself to enter into the world of non-doing.

Bring your attention inward by closing your eyes softly or rest the gaze in front of you leaving the eyelids just slightly open. Settle into this moment and begin to feel yourself sitting. You might notice these sensations from the inside out. Ride the movement of the breath as you breathe through the nose. Anchor in the breath wherever it meets your awareness most easily.

You might focus on the quiet hum vibrating through the body or the sensation of the breath at the belly. Wherever you meet the breath, let it carry in a gentle flow of energy, enlivening and awakening you to who you truly are—already whole.

By now, you may have noticed the thinking mind taking you away from the moment. Just begin to observe your inner experience of that distraction. And now, getting to know the mind well, let the spotlight of awareness begin to track the thoughts as bubbles on a stream. They arise, exist, and float away. For the next minute or so, be fully attentive to those thoughts, counting each of them as they move through.

Allow yourself to root in quiet stillness like a stone in the Ganges River. The water flowing all around you, at times turbulent with a stir of bubbles racing by, at other times a more peaceful current with only a bubble or two dancing along the surface.

Observe the thoughts with a friendly mind, an equanimous mind—just witnessing without reaction. Thoughts are neither good nor bad, right nor wrong. They're just thoughts. If the thoughts become too unsettling, you can always open your eyes for a moment.

And when you're ready, turn inward again and come back to counting the thoughts. Images, memories, inner stories, or the quiet whisper of words—all bubbles passing through. Planning, judging, arranging, more bubbles to count.

As you learn to allow the inner experience, without chasing or wishing those thought bubbles away, you begin to see a deeper truth. None of it is solid. To touch it lightly is to penetrate the skin and the bubble quickly disappears. But when you fight with the thoughts, you will find yourself in unending war. Allow each one. In time you'll begin to see those thoughts are all impermanent on the river of awareness. They arise, exist, and float away.

Breathe, notice, and be.

Awakening Our Dreams

TIME NEEDED: 9 MINUTES

THIS MEDITATION IS a guide to a deep and spacious inner listening. Here we'll welcome intentions and aspirations with the heart qualities that help manifest great potential.

Allow yourself to come into a comfortable position, finding stillness.

You might close your eyes if that's helpful.

And now bring your attention to the sensation of the breath wherever it meets your awareness.

You might sense the body breathing itself.

Bring in a sense of openness, a kind attention to whatever may be arising in this moment.

And now begin to draw your awareness to the intentions and desires you're bringing as you start this process of inner awakening. Notice the words that spring up naturally and reflect what you're calling into your life. Maybe you have the desire to feel more empowered. Self-accepting. Present. Just be aware of the words that come forward automatically and the ones that connect naturally with the heart. When it's right, you'll feel it. Calm. Steady. Fearless. Just letting yourself notice the qualities that you most hope to embody. Radiant. Joyful. Resilient. This is where we listen in to what really matters most. Connected. Open. Loving. Notice which words nourish you and bring you to life. Wrap them around you and see how they feel.

This journey is deeply personal, informed by your aspirations and your desires.

What you give your time and attention to serves as a compass for the direction of your life.

Today and each day of this practice, let yourself open into communication with your intuitive knowing, receiving and yielding to the truth of your wise inner voice. A fundamental strength of feminine consciousness is a profound capacity to manifest visions. Here we can use that gift to see clearly what we're calling into our lives.

At the end of this meditation, write your aspirations down. Then concentrate your attention on just a few. Get to know them well. Let yourself live with these words in the days to come. Henry David Thoreau once said, "Though I do not believe that a plant will spring up where there was no seed, I have great faith in a seed. Convince me you have a seed there, and I am prepared to expect wonders." May these words be the seeds that fill your soul and return you to this work again, and again.

Calm	Powerful	Passionate
Steady	Purposeful	Serene
Fearless	Present	Strengthened
Radiant	Courageous	Patient
Joyful	Authentic	Tolerant
Resilient	Empowered	Self-Accepting
Connected	Expressive	Peaceful
Open	Heart-Centered	Easy
Compassionate	Abundant	Free

Maya's Story: Afterword

Like many women I see, Maya had the life she'd carefully cultivated and claimed. It's the life she was told she should want. In truth, it was layered with a plethora of challenges: anxiety, insomnia, fatigue, irritability, and lately, severe migraines. Maya was suffering. She was lost in a life so informed by the agendas of others that she could no longer hear her true voice.

But no matter how lost we might be, our self-healing forces are always guiding us back. It often takes something intensely powerful to wake us up. For Maya, the intensity of her pain prompted her to take action, to take the brave step of going deeply inward with radical self-honesty. She then began the process of undoing, confronting, and releasing the patterns and expectations from family, partners, work colleagues, and culture itself. She examined the ways that she had participated and bought into the steady diet of striving and proving her worth. Maya looked hard at the ways she could support her well-being with practices to heal her mind-body system. And perhaps most importantly, she became her own advocate—coming home to her own heart and saying no to others a whole lot more in order to say yes to herself.

Top 3 Takeaways

1. Stress is a feminist issue. Culturally based stress and the impact it has on our mind-body is both a serious health risk to women and a cultural issue that can no longer be ignored.

2. Stress is not the enemy; in fact, life's obstacles can become our greatest gateways to awakening. Short-term stress bolsters our well-being and motivates us to reach farther than we thought possible. It's long-term, chronic stress that wreaks havoc on our health and happiness.

3. When we get to know our body and mind intimately, we can heal and empower ourselves in the face of chronic stress.

Journal Prompts

- In what ways do you believe the cultural messages you experience every day are having an impact on your life and overall well-being?

- In this chapter we introduced the notion of eustress, the helpful type of stress, which motivates and helps us build immunity. Think back over the past few years and recall a few times when short-term stress was healthy and perhaps even empowering for you. Think, too, about the hidden signs of chronic stress and write about ways your body is wisely asking (if not imploring) you to take notice.

- What do you notice in your body, your emotional tone, and your thinking mind as you connect deeply with the life you most want to live? What are your deepest intentions for this work? What impact do you hope it might make in your life? What inner quality will you meet the intention with?

2

Healing

Our Innate Ability
to Heal

*"Healing may not be so much about getting better as about
letting go of everything that isn't you—all of the expectations,
all of the beliefs—and becoming who you are."*

RACHEL NAOMI REMEN, Professor of Integrative Medicine, University of California

My Story

In 2018 I joined one of my favorite yoga teachers for a training session in Los Angeles. My mind needed a break, my body needed to
move, and my soul needed palm trees and warm sun. At least that's
what I told myself. We gathered, tuned in, and the yogic practice
began. However, put me in a class with thirty other people and all
intentions of relaxation and unity can get pushed aside. An internal
voice tells me, "If you're not pushing yourself harder than anyone
else, you're not trying." So while I hadn't been in a yoga class for over
six months, I still insisted on performing the best, deepest, most
enviable backbend of my twenty-year-long yoga practice. The end

result: a neck injury that brought me to my knees physically and emotionally for almost a year.

This win-at-all-costs mentality isn't a surprise given my upbringing on the North American race car circuit, where my father was a professional driver. To live as a "track rat" is to grow up in a world fueled by adrenaline. The smell of ethanol, the crowds clapping and cheering, the announcer yelling over the mic, my body in the clutches of both excitement and fear. Even today, when I visit that child in my mind, my heart quickens. I see her at the edge of the track praying hard and negotiating with God, "I'll be good, just let him win this race." And then the violent crashes. Screeching tires, confusion, race cars flying up in the air and turning over like toy cars, the crowd gasping, my mind crying out, "Please, don't let that be my dad's car."

The trauma to my neck (and vagus nerve) at the yoga retreat brought pain, blurred vision, migraines, and unrelenting anxiety. I eventually realized that my body was reacting not only to those memories but also to the fact that my childhood fears had been actualized a decade earlier when a car accident had left my dad paraplegic. Now my body was speaking, and life as I knew it was changing. With no place to hide, I had to start trusting and listening to the pain. I reached out to a team of healers (both allopathic and integrative) and scheduled peace talks with my mind-body. In time and with a whole lot of support, I learned to pay attention to the pain with a little more kindness. I began to open to the jolts and throbbing and seizing with less resistance. I began to trust that the breath would carry me through. And instead of wishing the sensations away, I surrendered to them as they arose, existed, and dissolved. Not always, but often enough.

And as I listened to the discomfort, I began to tend to that scared little girl, to visit her in my mind as I walked on the seawall or sat for a cup of tea. I invited her along and spoke with her, honored her courage, and freed her from fear.

Letting the Body and Mind Speak

So many of the stress-reduction methods proven to be effective in research studies just haven't resonated with the women I've worked with in counseling. While I'd explain the science and walk them through the techniques, these women would return the following week criticizing themselves for having failed to find the time to practice. But the problem wasn't a lack of effort or desire or capacity. The approaches themselves were the barrier. Instead of helping, the therapy was reinforcing the unconscious oppressive structures that women face every day. As I taught the protocols and mirrored the standardized language, they often felt unnatural and even awkward. The words lacked softness, felt removed and counterintuitive. These procedures resonated so poorly because they were laden with the masculine language of the men who developed them. Many of the relaxation techniques used today were born from the psychotherapeutic movement of the 1920s and the way they are delivered reflects the hierarchical dynamics of that era: directive, noncollaborative, and detached.

I wanted more for the women who were willing to entrust me with their well-being. I stopped using fancy language to mask my own insecurities, and we redesigned the approaches in ways that honored the feminine spirit. The exercises became less about performing and more about journeying inward and self-discovery. We dropped the measured goals and began to draw on the natural, intuitive wisdom of the feminine. We stopped talking and began listening. And we saw progress.

Biofeedback: Calm Body, Calm Mind

Stress is born from the mind's reaction to the events that unfold in our lives; it's highly subjective. Have you noticed that you can have the same experience as a friend or family member and have a completely different reaction? How we respond to a roller coaster, barking dog, presentation at work, and countless other events depends on internalized perceptions informed by our past experiences—and the body doesn't lie. Biofeedback is a practice of developing greater awareness of the many physiological responses of one's own body. We naturally shift and adjust at varied levels of consciousness all the time. At the heart of biofeedback is self-regulation: if we're out in the sun and we become hot, we drink water or move into the shade. If we're running and we can no longer catch our breath, we slow down. But stress can create an amazing discrepancy between what our body is experiencing as lived reality and how our mind is perceiving it. When we experience a steady stream of pressure, we're not always sensitive to the incremental changes. Just like the metaphor of a frog in slowly warming water failing to perceive the increasing danger, when stress levels rise gradually our signaling system can fail to alert us to "get out."

With some easy and intuitive biofeedback tools, we can tap into the body's subtle signals and sensations and increase our innate ability to self-regulate and consciously change the physical impact of stress on our mind-body system. When we allow our heart rate, blood flow, blood pressure, and other states of arousal to make their way out of the stress zone, we can harmonize the relationship between our mind, heart, and body. Then we feel greater ease and a relaxed core essence begins to shine through.

Relaxation techniques are a natural biofeedback method. They draw attention to the internal states of the mind-body system and signal the breath, muscles, blood flow, heart rate, and other functions in ways that return us to homeostasis, or equilibrium. All kinds of well-researched home-based biofeedback equipment programs are proven to support well-being. Whereas some focus on the relaxation response, others synchronize the nervous system and heart-brain frequency. The online biofeedback program called HeartMath,[1] for example, has over 300 independent peer-reviewed studies supporting its benefits. The program helps to change our heart rhythm from an erratic and disordered state of anxiety to a stable, smooth, and coherent pattern. Training the mind-body system to generate a better heart rhythm makes it a whole lot easier to calm the body, emotions, and thinking mind.

Ujjayi Pranayama (Ocean Breath)

TIME NEEDED: 6 MINUTES

IT WILL PROBABLY come as no surprise that the regular practice of controlled breathing has such a naturally healing impact on our mind-body system—after all, breathing is living. And while you'll find a whole chapter (see chapter 5) dedicated to its wondrous role in our overall health, we'll start to use it here as part of our biofeedback practice. Breath is the ultimate biofeedback method. It directly calms the nervous system and soothes the agitated mind.

Listen to your breath and follow me in this exercise called Ujjayi Pranayama (Ocean Breath), the ancient Hindu practice of breath control that is the foundation of yoga. The goal of Ujjayi Pranayama is to strengthen the connection between body and mind by focusing attention on the breath, expanding the lungs, and consciously attending to the ocean sound as you inhale and exhale.

Let's begin.

Sit comfortably on the floor with legs crossed or on a firm chair. Lengthen the spine and bring the chin slightly down. Now breathe in slowly until you reach your lungs' full capacity, hold your breath for a moment, then release the breath constricting some of the breath at the back of the throat. Exhale slowly and listen to the gentle release of air—it may sound like the ocean's waves. As you exhale, see if you can feel the air at the roof of the mouth and the back of the throat. Keep repeating, fully expanding the lungs with each inhale and exhaling with a gentle rush of air.

When you become distracted, just return to the sound—the light hiss of the breath. With each breath be fully present to each sensation, each emotion, and thought. Know it for the moment and let it go. Expand the lungs with each breath. Always return to the breath. If you experience any discomfort, just breathe into the discomfort with tolerance and patience. Trust that the body knows what to do. Let each breath be gentle and controlled.

With every inhale, receive this new moment. With each exhale, let go of whatever came before. Your breath is always present, constantly available, faithfully returning you to the unending now. It asks only that you notice.

Breathe, notice, and be.

___

LISTENING TO OUR HANDS (FEET)

Are you listening to what your hands are telling you? Have you ever noticed that it can be hot and sunny out and yet your hands are cold? Our hands (and feet) tell us so much more than we often realize about the state of our mind-body system. When our nervous system is in chronic overdrive, the mind and body work together to put protective systems in place. An increase in the stress hormone adrenaline triggers a change in blood flow away from the feet and hands and toward the core to safeguard the organs from danger. The result is icy cold extremities. And while cold hands can be related to other conditions, they may be signaling that our nervous system is in fight-or-flight mode. While the blood flows toward the core, our heart rate increases and our muscles tense. Our body's encoded wisdom suppresses immune function and the rest-and-repair response so it can mobilize the energy we might need to protect us from harm.

In contrast, have you noticed how soothing it feels to hold a warm hand, slip into a pair of fuzzy slippers, or wrap your fingers around a warm cup of tea? The hands and feet are sending important signals to the brain and activating the parasympathetic (calming) nervous system. In part, the comfort is coming from the primal brain. Blood flowing toward the hands and feet signals safety. But the brain-body axis is bidirectional. With specific relaxation techniques we can begin to use the power of the mind to purposefully direct the blood flow to the hands and feet, raising our skin temperature and calming the mind, heart, and body.

AUTOGENIC TRAINING

In the 1920s, German psychotherapist Johannes Heinrich Schultz established a method he called autogenic training. It was an innovative approach to helping patients relax by having them regulate their breath while directing blood flow to the hands and feet through muscle relaxation. He taught his patients to use the power of their mind to imagine their extremities warming, and their body cooperated. Over the past hundred years the approach has been investigated widely, with reviews showing it to be effective for relieving conditions such as tension headaches, hypertension, pain disorders, panic disorders, sleep disorders, depression, Raynaud's disease, and more.[2] And for anxiety specifically, the evidence for autogenic training is indisputable, with meta-analysis studies (the gold standard of science) showing it to significantly reduce symptoms of anxiety.[3]

Autogenic Training
(Return to Calm)

TIME NEEDED: 9 MINUTES

THE FOLLOWING AUTOGENIC training practice was recreated from Schultz's original version to help calm the body and soothe the over-active mind, all through the heart of the feminine.

If you'd like to be scientific about this, pick up a stress ther-mometer (you can find them online) and write down your skin temperature before and after doing the biofeedback exercises in this chapter. Doing the exercise at the same time and in the same room each day can bolster the accuracy. If the science doesn't interest you, simply follow the process daily (or when time allows) and notice its impact. Try these practices with a curious mind and in time you'll curate a collection of health practices that are uniquely honoring and effective for you.

Before you begin, find a comfortable and quiet place to lie down and relax. Remove your glasses and cozy up with a warm blanket. If you're using a temperature sensor, rest your hands easily outside the blanket.

Allow the eyelids to gently close and the body to become still. Close your eyes if you like and let your inner gaze and stillness return you fully to this moment, right here, right now.

Bring your attention to the rhythm of the breath as you breathe through the nose. Let the breath trace the path of a rolling hill, rising on the in-breath and falling on the out-breath. Gently slow the breath, rising for a count of 1, 2, 3, 4, 5 and falling for 5, 4, 3, 2, 1.

Let the breath restore you to the peace of this moment as it coaxes out the fear from places deep within. Feel it move through the body as you whisper, "I am here, and I am calm."

Let the body feel the earth cradling it with unwavering care as you release the hold of the day. And may you find yourself in this rest.

Notice the sensations at the arms. Arms heavy. The left arm is heavy. The right arm is heavy. Both of the arms are heavy.

Repeating these words: "I am here, and I am calm."

Bringing full attention now to the legs. Notice the sensations there. The legs, too, begin to find stillness. Legs are heavy. The left leg is heavy. The right leg is heavy. Both of the legs are heavy.

Repeating these words: "I am here, and I am calm."

Let the mind dream of sun and sand and a healing warmth running its current through your tired bones. The heat tracing a path to the hands, blowing life, like a wise woman's breath, on frosty fingers.

Notice the sensations at the hands. Hands are warm. The left hand is warm. The right hand is warm. Both hands are warm.

Repeating these words: "I am here, and I am calm."

With each inhale and exhale you are soothed and restored and warmed to your bones. Like campfire sticks, the wise woman rubs her hands together and places them against your icy feet. Her body heats yours.

Bring attention to the feet and notice any sensations there—anything that is there to be felt. Feet are warm. The left foot is warm. The right foot is warm. Both feet are warm.

Repeating these words: "I am here, and I am calm."

The abdomen rises and falls, swells and recedes, soothed in the intimacy of it all. The forehead cools and the mind sees. You place the hand at the heart center. Heartbeat steady, body warm and heavy.

Repeating these words: "I am here, and I am calm, and may it always be so."

Breathe, notice, and be.

A LITTLE NOTE OF ENCOURAGEMENT

It's OK to feel awkward. The pathway back to ourselves and our well-being can feel both mysterious and uncomfortable, a process we're asked to trust but don't fully understand. It's this enigmatic quality that often holds people back from opening the gateway to self-realization or continuing when progress slows or regresses. Transformation occurs in phases. Although they may dance in different positions in your own healing journey, here are some stages of self-realization you can expect along the way.

The Call for Change: You feel so disconnected from your true self that you're ready to do whatever it takes to create change.

Inception: You discover the innate healer that will walk alongside you and guide you into the shadows so that you may face the fears and parts suppressed deep within.

The Dark Night: You begin to touch the pain and fear and anger you've kept tucked away deep inside, and as you do the emotions may intensify. You learn to meet the discomfort with greater openness and patience.

The Opening: As you metabolize the old pain patterns and practice new tools to open to the changing flow of experience, the sirens are reduced to whispers of discomfort and you begin to feel a lightness from within.

The True Self: You can better hear the voice of the true self, the essence of who you really are. You can observe the irrational beliefs of the thinking mind more easily and you know that you are not those beliefs. You can now shed the limitations and illusions of who you thought you once were.

Integration: You begin to see your life anew, filled with possibility. You're clear about what serves you, supports you, and what needs to be released in order to live in your highest well-being.

Higher Purpose: You are awakened to a greater consciousness—the formless awareness that is our source. Your heart is no longer armored, and you have a strength of spirit that guides you into the current of your higher purpose. Your gifts are untethered, and you feel deep in your bones that your life is meaningful beyond measure.

Keep in mind that the process of healing and transformation is not at all linear. You may find yourself in one stage of self-realization and then feel hurled back into a more uncomfortable previous one. It's then that you may want to throw in the towel (or destroy this book altogether), but that's exactly when breakthroughs often emerge. The most important advice I can offer is to keep going! Recommit to yourself again and again and again. In time, the practices designed to support you will feel more natural and you'll feel less like Bambi on ice.

Relax into Healing

Progressive muscle relaxation (PMR) has been used to release stress and foster well-being for over 100 years. The technique was originally developed by the American psychiatrist Edmund Jacobson as a step-by-step way to calm the body and mind. Jacobson was one of the first modern psychiatrists to acknowledge the interrelationship between mind and body, and he was fascinated by the connection between excessive muscular tension and both physical and mental illness. He dedicated his life to investigating the relationship between tension, muscle tone, and the impact on the central nervous system. His seminal book, *You Must Relax*, remains one of the most important books in somatic psychotherapy.[4]

Since Jacobson's time, PMR has been shown to bring very real and lasting changes to the health of our mind-body system. During PMR, the muscle groups are systematically stretched and relaxed to promote blood flow and lymphatic flow, decrease blood pressure, improve organ function, and support the health of the muscles and connective tissues. It's like an internal massage.[5]

In one study, PMR was shown to be a remarkable source of solace for hospital patients suffering from COVID-19. Those who were taught the technique from nurses felt less anxious and slept better.[6] Imagine if this practice can soothe fear for those facing a life-threatening disease what it may offer you as you weave these new threads of well-being.

Progressive Muscle Relaxation

TIME NEEDED: 24 MINUTES

PROGRESSIVE MUSCLE RELAXATION is an inner process to guide the mind-body system back to its natural state of well-being. During each step of this practice, allow the body to lead you into places that need your attention. Allow resistance, discomfort, difficult emotion, and any unpleasant sensation to arise without pushing against it or judging the experience as good or bad, right or wrong. Let it be so. If you experience pleasant sensations like relief or elation, simply notice what may be arising without chasing or craving more. Again, let it be so. This equanimous approach will allow you to experience the moment more fully without wishing it to be different.

Essential oils, such as lavender and jasmine, can deepen the body's relaxation response and draw the mind into a meditative state.[7] Consider using a diffuser to support your daily practices.

Find a quiet place to rest and turn the lights down low. Feel the hum of energy running through the body as you rest against a chair or lie on the floor or in bed. Allow yourself to open to the life that is unfolding with you, for you. You are right at the doorway; you need only step into the current of this healing practice. Here you may rest, replenish, restore, and strengthen. When you notice the mind wander, guide it back to the way of the body and breath.

Breathe through the nose and draw in a long, low, slow breath, hold for a moment, and then exhale gently and settle into this practice. There is no better use of time today than this. You might imagine cradling the breath—not holding it too firmly or too lightly.

Bring awareness now to the sensation at the feet. Gently stretch the feet and wiggle the toes, awakening them with gratitude for holding you strong as you move through this wondrous life. Toes draw upward, reaching their way as if to fully receive the grace of your attention. Reaching for 5, 4, 3, 2, 1, and rest. Notice the difference between the tension and relaxation. Again, drawing the toes up for 5, 4, 3, 2, 1, and rest.

Repeating these words inwardly, "I am grateful for these feet and these toes."

Bring awareness to the sensation at the legs. Feeling now the strength of the legs as you scan your awareness from ankle to hip. Notice now those forgotten places within, the places of holding and tension, openness and ease. Remember now all the times those legs held you steady. Begin to contract calf and thigh, squeezing and releasing that which is ready to release for 5, 4, 3, 2, 1, and rest. Notice the difference between the tension and relaxation. Again, 5, 4, 3, 2, 1, and rest.

Repeating these words inwardly, "I am grateful for these legs."

Bring awareness to the sensation at the hands. The hands humming with the way of touch, of tenderness, of creation. Allow one hand to meet the other touching lightly and feeling the aliveness as the fingertips roll across the skin. Begin to squeeze the hands with great might, releasing now any frustration or anger or rage that may be held deep within those muscles and bones for 5, 4, 3, 2, 1, and rest. Notice the difference now. Again, 5, 4, 3, 2, 1, and rest.

Repeating these words inwardly, "I am grateful for these hands."

Bring awareness to the sensation at the arms. Beautiful are these arms that hold and embrace your dear ones. Held open, they mend bruised hearts and offer a loving abyss and refuge from the swirling eddies of sorrow. Bring the palm up toward the shoulder and now squeeze both arms, bringing your fullest attention to the task, for 5, 4, 3, 2, 1, and rest. Notice the difference, notice the sensation. Again, 5, 4, 3, 2, 1, and rest.

Repeating these words inwardly, "I am grateful for these arms."

Bring awareness to the sensation at the belly. Place the hands against the belly and bring to mind all those times you may have held the emotions of others, denied what you intuitively knew was right, or ignored your need for sustenance. Know that you did your best with what you understood at that time. Contract the belly, releasing anything you might be holding there, for 5, 4, 3, 2, 1, and rest. Noticing now any sensation. Again, 5, 4, 3, 2, 1, and rest.

Repeating these words inwardly, "I am grateful for this belly."

Bring awareness to the sensation at the hips. Be aware of the hips, round and curved they speak your power and worth and spirited ways. Squeeze the hips now as if to hug hard the seat of the feminine, holding tight with admiration for it all. 5, 4, 3, 2, 1, and rest. Just notice. Again, 5, 4, 3, 2, 1, and rest.

Repeating these words inwardly, "I am grateful for these hips."

Bring awareness to the sensation at the mouth. Notice the softness of the mouth. Your wise words soothe the brokenhearted, calm fear, strengthen boundaries, and stop hatred in its tracks. Squeeze the lips together, enlivening and inviting the release of anything that prevents you from speaking what is true for you, for 5, 4, 3, 2, 1, and rest. And notice. Again, 5, 4, 3, 2, 1, and rest.

Repeating these words inwardly, "I am grateful for this mouth."

Bring awareness to the sensation at the heart. Sink into the heart center, giving yourself fully to the healing power of the heart. Allowing yourself to be steadied by its rhythm. The heart guides you on your darkest days; it is your true home. Wrap your arms around the body, hugging tightly through the heart center, disarming any barriers to feeling fully as you squeeze for 5, 4, 3, 2, 1, and rest. Notice the sensation now. Again, 5, 4, 3, 2, 1, and rest.

Repeating these words inwardly, "I am grateful for this heart."

Bring awareness to the sensation at the eyes. Notice now the shadows dancing behind the eyelids, casting form, reflecting each unfolding moment of life. These windows to this wondrous world show you the ways of joy and pain, love and longing, all of life's hues just as they are. Hold the eyes tight as you squeeze any tension away for 5, 4, 3, 2, 1, and rest. Noticing the difference. Again, 5, 4, 3, 2, 1, and rest.

Repeating these words inwardly, "I am grateful for these eyes."

Bring awareness to the sensation at the neck. Noticing any current of emotion running through. Take a moment to feel into the emotional tension that hides and hibernates there. Draw great kindness into this area of holding and squeeze chin to neck for 5, 4, 3, 2, 1, and rest. Right ear to shoulder, 5, 4, 3, 2, 1, and rest. Left ear to shoulder for 5, 4, 3, 2, 1, and rest. Notice the difference between tension and relaxation.

Repeating these words inwardly, "I am grateful for this neck."

Bring awareness to the sensation at the shoulders. The shoulders are the resting place of worry and burdens known and unknown. Lift the shoulders up to the ears, releasing all that you've held and hidden away for 5, 4, 3, 2, 1, and rest. Notice the subtle difference. Again, 5, 4, 3, 2, 1, and rest.

Repeating these words inwardly, "I am grateful for these shoulders."

Bring awareness to the sensation at the forehead and the third eye, resting in living presence. Now lift the eyebrows high to the sky, reaching and releasing for 5, 4, 3, 2, 1, and rest. Notice the sensation now. Again, 5, 4, 3, 2, 1, and rest.

Feel the current of peace as it runs through the entire body as you repeat these words inwardly, "I am grateful for this body, this breath, and this life. I am here now and I am at peace."

My Story: Afterword

I journeyed through meditation, wrote page after page of dreams and memories and emotions long ignored. I turned to acupuncture and somatic psychotherapy, and gave myself permission to rest physically, mentally, and emotionally. Nature was my medicine. With each walk in the forest I felt more restored, connected, and whole again. I learned to slooooow down and judge myself (and my body) a little less. As my mind and body healed, my heart felt softer and I felt more present and open to both the pain and the joy. The injury that had taken me into terror served me well. It helped me break through the self-protective layers of trauma and delivered me back to my true self.

Top 3 Takeaways

1. Our innate ability to self-heal is miraculous. To leverage that ability, we need to learn the ways of listening to our body and mind.

2. We can carry the past in the body but it doesn't have to inform our life. We have the capacity to metabolize the conditions from the past, freeing ourselves from its impact.

3. Relaxation techniques act as a natural biofeedback method, drawing attention to the mind-body system and signaling the breath, muscles, blood flow, heart rate, and other functions in ways that return us to the calm conditions that allow us to experience life openly and fully.

Journal Prompts

- As you begin to listen to the messages of the body, exploring and feeling deeply the sensations it's communicating (both subtle and intense), what are you discovering?

- What would it be like to witness the discomfort a little longer and remain with the body when it needs you the most?

- What are you not allowing yourself to feel?

- Take some time to write a love letter to your body, asking that it forgive you for all the times you held it to unreasonable and harmful standards. And know that you did the very best that you could at that time.

- Every time you return to the body you're rooting into the vessel of your soul. What would be different in your life if you took time throughout each day to pause, return to the body, open to what's there, and offer loving support through the breath and tools you now have?

Meditation

A Gateway to Well-Being

*"You must learn to be still in the midst of activity
and to be vibrantly alive in repose."*

INDIRA GANDHI

Jen's Story

Jen is a fierce feeler, openhearted and authentic in a way that feels beautifully honest. When others hurt, she hurts, which is not an easy path in a culture with so much pain. When she came to see me, she had been working at a relentless pace in a tech start-up company for over a year. Her doctor had prescribed various medications to treat anxiety, but any improvement was negligible. The anxiety was literally making her sick: she felt nauseous, and she was sleep deprived and living in fear. She had reached her limits and her body's alarm systems were ringing so loudly that she could no longer hear her own voice. To Jen, the anxiety felt permanent and debilitating, and like most clients in her situation she was eager to see how meditation and other mind-body health practices might help relieve the distress.

We talked about the mind-body connection and how certain approaches to meditation can help soothe anxiety. I asked her to let go of any expectations about or conditions for meditation and be open to whatever the practice wanted to show her. We weren't looking to create a "new and improved" version of Jen, but to guide her toward self-healing and a path to her true self.

At first, Jen found meditation counterintuitive and almost impossible. While she began to see very clearly what was happening in her anxious mind, her sense of groundlessness intensified as she opened to it. She would squirm and resist, and I would gently remind her that the mind wanders, tells stories, and amplifies the fear and drama because that's what the mind does. She learned to meet the thoughts with less reaction, and bit by bit she guided her attention back to the sensation of the breath. In time, she became still enough for long enough to witness the sensations of fear and distress with more compassion and awareness. She recognized that every breath was an opportunity to face the emotions she had been avoiding, and the more often she relaxed, the more easily she could detach from the emotional pain and physical discomfort.

Jen became kinder to herself. She attuned to the sensations in her body and watched her mind go down the pathways of fear, uncertainty, and guilt and engage in mundane mind chatter without adding more layers of story. She became more curious about what her body was telling her and learned to detach from anxiety by opening to the sensations. She learned to label the chatter as "thinking." That's what we do in meditation: we learn to drop the stories and accept the moment as it is, without craving for it to be different. In this way, we observe and see clearly the patterns of thinking and feeling that we've replayed over and over again. In time, we drop the attachment to the egoic mind and we awaken to our remarkable, ordinary lives.

As Jen learned to listen deeply to a wiser part of herself, she began to shape her life in ways that honored her desire for greater meaning.

She left her job in tech and went back to school to study therapy so that she could help and heal and support others. And while meditation was not a cure for pain or pleasure or the pace of life itself, she discovered a way to respect and listen to the wisdom within her.

Becoming Wholeheartedly Ourselves

By learning to observe the changing nature of our mind and body we have the potential to gain a profound and life-changing self-knowledge, a deep inner knowing that can lead to enduring peace. Is facing the unruly mind sometimes daunting? Yes. But in time we begin to see the impermanent flow of thought, emotion, sensation, and the unfolding of our lives with greater compassion and a little more humor. We tend to take our human predicament very seriously at times!

Most of the time we're asleep at the wheel, but meditation gives us a chance to free the mind from the unconscious conditions that remove us from the present moment. The longer we sit in stillness and silence, using these ancient and codified systems of training the mind, the more proficient we become at meeting life exactly where it is. Between surges of discomfort emerge moments when thoughts are transcended, the mind recedes, and we begin to discover the magic of unbroken awareness. The present becomes expansive. We feel an inner spaciousness more often, and from that spaciousness comes a natural radiance of joy and goodness. Every time we meditate, we have the potential to open a gateway to the awe and wonder of life itself, to embrace all of it.

Meditation isn't about making ourselves different or better—there is no improving the perfect essence of who we are already. It's about being the fullest version of ourselves. Bringing a wakefulness and kindness to our relationship with ourselves is a beautiful thing. I believe that if each of us chooses to sit in quiet contemplation each day, every day, we have the capacity not only to awaken to our true selves but also to elevate the wakefulness required to support our planet's survival.

Meditation is an ongoing process of ever-increasing awareness, and what we practice on the mat prepares us to face our lives with greater wisdom. And what we repeat, we embody. Meditation primes the brain for calm, focused awareness and the heart for compassion beyond measure. It changes first our state (the heart rate decreases, feelings of restful alertness increase, and the thinking mind settles) and then our enduring traits (improved resiliency to stress, greater compassion for ourselves and others, better focused attention, and we become less self-absorbed).[1] It is a training ground for a kinder, wiser way.

While meditation allows us to open up, that doesn't mean that when we sit, close our eyes, and turn inward, we always find bliss. The discomfort and steady stream of thoughts don't magically go away. Meditation shows us exactly where we're opening up or shutting down, trying to escape or leaning in. There's no running away. Meditation is a mirror with acute accuracy, and no matter how the mirror is angled, we see ourselves exactly as we are. We come face-to-face with our disappointment, anger, sadness, resentment, pain, and anxiety. We see clearly all the ways we manipulate the moment, amplifying, avoiding, or entertaining ourselves with fantasies and wishes. Meditation teaches us to stop struggling and soften into ourselves.

The effects of meditation are gradual and cumulative. The neurobiological changes that occur with every minute of contemplative practice make it one of the most potent and trusted ways to expand well-being. A research group at Johns Hopkins University reviewed almost 19,000 meditation studies and included forty-seven randomized clinical trials.[2] They found that regular meditation had an overwhelming ability to quell anxiety and relieve symptoms of depression and pain (among many other benefits).

Not all meditation approaches are alike, however. Contemplative practices, for example, are a training ground, a mental gym where we can exercise the parts of the brain that help regulate the thoughts and emotions that pull us out of the moment.[3] And if we want to strengthen our emotional stability, self-awareness, and focused attention (who doesn't?!), then contemplative meditation may be the answer.[4] For greater self-compassion, connection, or altruism, Metta meditation (also known as loving-kindness meditation) is well proven to get us there.[5] Certain mindfulness practices have also been shown to reduce pain and leave meditators less emotionally reactive to it when it arises.[6]

Maitri

So often meditation becomes another focal point for self-criticism because we decide we're not doing it properly or not practicing frequently enough. We turn inward, try to settle into the body, and then come the judgment, self-criticism, and barrage of fear-based thoughts we've been trying so hard to avoid. When we scold ourselves for not meditating correctly, this practice becomes just another way to reinforce the same old mind patterns. But we don't meditate to perfect meditation; we do it to awaken to our lives.

Imagine meditating with an attitude of *maitri*, the Buddhist term for "loving kindness." The transformative impact of maitri is perhaps one of the most important and overlooked conditions of meditation. As we practice opening more gently to what's there, we prune the brain's established patterns and reshape the mind for calm, compassionate awareness. Maitri doesn't mean that we deny or sugarcoat reality: quite the opposite. It asks us to look clearly at what is meeting our field of awareness without amplifying it, obsessing over it, or adding a story to what's there. With maitri we look at ourselves in a very direct way and we address what we see with curiosity and even humor.

Retraining the mind for maitri can take a lifetime of practice, but small steps lead to radical shifts in well-being. As you begin your meditation practice, take a moment to settle into your heart center by placing the hand at the heart. Practice with a half-smile and allow the corners of the eyes to reach up to the sky, calling in maitri. Honor your practice by speaking your intention for openness out loud. When I teach a meditation group, I often suggest that we harmonize with the wish "May I keep an open heart and mind so I may see what is there to be seen, heal what is there to be healed, and come home to who I am in truth." We also dedicate our contemplative practice to the betterment of all beings, acknowledging our interconnectedness.

Meditation Has Something for Everyone

Although meditation has been a part of Eastern spiritual traditions for centuries, its primary purpose has never been to help us relax, improve our focus, or sleep better. Any benefits such as these are secondary to the true goal of developing a deep contemplative process and an awakened quality of being. As we've adapted meditation to Western culture, we have borrowed some traditions while leaving others behind. We have emphasized guided short-term practice in hopes of alleviating stress and other more immediate benefits. The kind of meditation I'm encouraging here is neither the deep path that comes with monastic dedication nor the user-friendly app-only version but something in between. And while your motivation for meditating may vacillate between the simple hope of feeling calmer and renewed and a deeper desire to discover true peace and freedom, know that the approach you use and the number of hours in practice matter if you're looking for lifelong change.[7]

The science and data on meditation are starting to reveal what works for whom and why. Many neuroscientists, physicists, and psychologists have committed their professional lives to this understanding and they are just now discovering the payoffs meditation brings to our physical health, mental well-being, and social connections. Scientific scholars are confirming what wisdom teachers have suspected all along: meditation changes the architecture of the mind in ways that can transform our well-being. Meditation may seem mystical since it was born from spiritual tradition, but the practice is accessible, its effectiveness borne out by rigorous scientific studies. Meditation is available to everyone, anywhere, any time.

8 THINGS YOU MIGHT NOT KNOW ABOUT MEDITATION

Still thinking of meditation as just a way to unwind after a long day? The benefits of meditation extend far beyond relaxation. Here are just some of the ways that meditation has been shown to support well-being:

1. Meditation helps to reduce symptoms of attention-deficit/hyperactivity disorder (ADHD). It's no surprise that meditation helps us focus, but we now know that it actually helps adults and adolescents with ADHD. In a 2008 study published in the *Journal of Attention Disorders*, 78% of participants reported a reduction in their symptoms after meditation.[8]

2. In patients with heart disease, meditation reduces the risk of heart attack and stroke. Patients who meditated for 20 minutes a day were less stressed and experienced a reduced risk of "endpoint cardiovascular events" as compared to a control group that did not meditate.[9]

3. Meditation increases social connection and emotional intelligence. A study showed that by increasing positive emotions, meditation produced feelings of increased purpose in life and social support, which led to an increase in life satisfaction and reduced depressive symptoms.[10]

4. Even a brief meditation session helps to improve our working memory and reduces fatigue. It's well established that meditating for longer periods of time produces cognitive benefits, but we now know that as few as four brief meditation sessions can improve mood and working memory.[11]

5. Meditation can improve analytical and problem-solving abilities. A 2015 study published in *Frontiers of Psychology* showed that mindful participants performed better when instructed to solve problems analytically than a control group made up of less mindful participants.[12]

6. Meditation enhances our creativity. Even for beginners, studies show that meditation techniques improve creative-thinking abilities and have lasting cognitive benefits.[13]

7. Meditation can improve our sex life. In a 2011 study, women who meditated were more able to register and attend to their own physiological responses to sexual stimuli, improving their libido and reducing symptoms of sexual dysfunction.[14]

8. Meditation may make our brain bigger and mitigate the effects of aging. In one study, the brain scans of long-term meditators showed thicker gray matter, even in older individuals, compared with non-meditators. The study's findings suggest that meditation is associated with cortical thickening and plasticity in the areas of the brain related to cognitive and emotional processing and well-being.[15]

A LITTLE NOTE OF ENCOURAGEMENT

Mindfulness, to pause and become aware, takes but a moment. We practice on the mat what we'd like to embody in everyday life, but it's possible to experience full awareness at any moment, no matter what we're doing. Cue the sacred pause. When we pause, we can pay attention, without judgment, to whatever exists in the moment—this is meditation. Tying the pause to a specific time or event makes it easier to remember. You might pause after each Zoom meeting, or after you go to the bathroom, or between conversations or activities to mark the transition. Take a moment now. Pause, become aware, notice the breath, and let go of the doing self. Relax the need to be anywhere else but here. Reconnect instead with the mystery of this moment.

ACKNOWLEDGING THE IMPORTANCE OF EXPECTATIONS

One of the greatest barriers to meditation is the expectation that closing the eyes will automatically lead to a feeling of bliss. This is not meditation. Although you may experience wonderful feelings and sensations while meditating, strong and painful thoughts and emotions can come up too. If the emotions become too "hot," open your eyes gently and return to the breath or whatever roots you into the body. In time, the mind learns to perceive these emotions without judgment and reactivity. For a small percentage of people, meditation can heighten mental health symptoms. If this happens, it's important to work with a meditation teacher and your health professional.

INVITATION TO PRACTICE: MASTERING POSTURE

The Buddha within you doesn't care if you sit on the floor, on a chair, or on the bus—although the bus may be a challenge for beginning meditators! Find a consistent and quiet place to sit each day. The mind creates patterns of association, so if you pair a certain place with meditation it strengthens the likelihood of a consistent practice.

Here are some tips for sitting during a meditation practice:

- Sit comfortably on a flat surface.

- Lengthen the spine, keeping the core sturdy yet relaxed.

- If sitting on a chair, position the body away from the backrest and keep the knees an inch or so apart.

- Bring the chin slightly down.

- Place the hands comfortably on the legs, palms down.

- Soften the shoulders, forehead, eyelids, and jaw, and place the tongue gently at the palate against the top teeth.

SETTING AN INTENTION

Connecting with the core intention we bring to the practice helps to clarify the reason for recommitting over and over again. If we don't clearly understand why we're in practice, it becomes harder to justify. When you set your intention, touch it lightly and then let it go. Let it fall away. When we hold fast to the intention or judge our experience because it's not in line with what we most wanted, we reinforce the conditions we're trying to free ourselves from. Whether we call in calm, more loving presence, greater focus, or strength in difficult times, we must be open to the guiding current of awareness. Let the meditation unfold as it wishes and show you what is there to be seen. When starting a meditation practice, it can be helpful to keep a journal to reflect on what you're discovering. Write about what you noticed in the mind and body during your practice, and explore your thoughts and feelings about any realizations, distractions, cravings and aversions, discomforts, barriers and supports. The meditation journal is meant to support your inner knowing, so be kind to yourself. If you're getting tripped up with perfectionism or judging and criticizing the length of your sit, level of distraction, or quality of your attention, simply return to the intention of equanimity and compassion.

DISCOVERING YOUR ANCHOR

An anchor is a point of focus that returns us to embodied awareness again and again. It faithfully returns us to the present moment when the mind wanders away. The anchor should feel natural, like a good dance partner. If you're new to meditation, explore which anchors are most supportive and then commit to mastering just one. Choose the one that steadies you most easily.

- To discover your anchor, start by closing your eyes and begin to attune to the breath.

- Breathe through the nose and let each breath bring you more fully into this moment.

- Follow the sensation of the in-breath and out-breath as it moves through the nostrils, or just below the nostril at the upper lip.

- If breathing through the nose is difficult, connect with the breath where it feels more natural.

- Feel its wave swell at the belly.

- Or follow the breath as it ripples through the body.

- Watch and witness as the body breathes itself.

- You can also combine the breath sensation with other physical sensations, like tingling in the hands.

- Or sensations at the third eye (the middle of the forehead).

- Your anchor might be the sounds as they enter your awareness.

- Choose whatever sensation opens you to your fullest presence.

COMING FACE-TO-FACE WITH SELF-CRITICISM

When we're making important changes in our lives, barriers have a way of showing themselves and making the flow of transformation just a little stickier. In most cases, these barriers are old internal patterns that the egoic mind isn't ready to give up. The egoic mind might tell you that you don't have enough time or the right meditation space, or that you're not capable of practicing successfully (whatever successful meditation means). One of the main barriers to committing to meditation practice is the relentless stream of self-criticism. We sit down, close our eyes, anchor in our breath, and the mind wanders to unanswered emails or an argument with our partner. When we realize we've lost our focus, we judge ourselves. When you recognize the mind has wandered, celebrate; it's in the noticing that you've awakened to the moment. And as for those distracting thoughts, observe them with compassion rather than wishing them away. Soften at the heart center and allow those thoughts to arise, exist, and pass through. You might breathe in some space between you and those thoughts and even giggle a little at the mind's neurotic tendencies. In time, the judging mind will settle. This is the detachment that comes with sustained practice.

DEALING WITH DISTRACTION, FEAR, BOREDOM, SLEEPINESS, AND PAIN

Everything that arises as you meditate is an opportunity to practice mindful awareness. If distraction surfaces, simply label it as "thinking" or "distraction." Notice what distraction feels like in the body and return to your anchor.

If fear comes up, label it as "fear" and allow yourself to be curious about the sensations. Connect to the heart center and talk to the fear compassionately. Say to the fear, "I've got you. Thank you for trying to protect me, but we're all good here." Then return to the breath. Or bring to mind the image of a spiritual guide or someone who supports you. Allow them to sit with you until the sensation of fear subsides.

If you become bored or sleepy, shift the body so you become more alert. You may be sleepy because the body is just plain tired or because the stillness of meditation signals to the body that it's time to sleep. It may also be a defense mechanism to keep the body from experiencing difficult or suppressed emotions. Whatever the reason, observe the boredom or sleepiness with compassion and let the judgment go. You might even ask, "What else am I feeling other than sleepy?"

Bring the same equanimity to sensations of pain. Calmly breathe into those sensations and notice your reaction to them. Do you meet emotional and physical pain with resentment, avoidance, or fear? Give the discomfort some loving kindness and return to your anchor.

Consciousness allows us to integrate our internal thoughts and feelings with our physical sensations. As we open to all that arises through the mind and body without reacting or pushing against it, we begin to observe, detach, and let go of the years of inner patterning. This practice leads to self-realization, and self-realization leads to freedom.

Anapanasati (Anchoring in the Breath)

TIME NEEDED: 16 MINUTES

ONE OF THE simplest and most effective ways to anchor into the moment is through anapanasati, the ancient Buddhist practice of mindfully observing the breath. *Anapana* refers to the "inhale and exhale" and *sati* means "mindfulness." Anapanasati is one of the most accessible and inclusive approaches to mind-body health we have available. After all, breath is common to all, free, and available anywhere and any time.

Find a comfortable place to sit. You might sit cross-legged on the floor or on a chair with a straight spine. Any position that supports an awake and dignified presence works well.

Let's take a moment to turn inward. You might close your eyes completely or shut the eyelids slightly as though you were adjusting the shutters of a window.

Rest in stillness and bring a relaxed openness to this moment.

Let the face be soft.

Relax the shoulders.

Allow the muscles to release the tension you've collected.

Enter gently into the world of non-doing.

This is a time to give to yourself fully.

Breathe, naturally, in and out through the nose if you can, and let each breath lift you from the weight of the day.

Just notice the breath as it enters the body and as it leaves the body.

Watch and witness the incoming breath and the outgoing breath.

This may be the first time all day that you notice the breath at all.

If you're not able to breathe through the nose, notice the sensation at the belly as it expands and subsides. Or you might feel the breath as it hums or radiates through the entire body.

All you're doing is simply tracking the breath.

With each inhale, relax into each new moment. And with each exhale, let go of whatever came before. The breath is always there, constantly available, faithfully returning you to the present. It asks only that you notice.

The breath makes its way to you so effortlessly.

Just let the breath come to you.

Lighting the path to present time.

The unending moment-to-moment reality.

No past and no future to worry about.

Just full and loving awareness of this ordinary and miraculous moment.

You might have a sense of witnessing the body breathing itself.

Or you might imagine yourself being breathed.

The breath entering the body and leaving the body.

Here there is no gaining, no striving, no seeking, and no proving your worth.

Meditation is not about being better or changing yourself.

It's a return to the truth that you are already whole.

Drop any effort and soften into the moment.

Right here, right now.

Observing life as it is.

The mind has probably taken you away many times already.

The thinking mind takes us into memories, planning, worrying, judging.

Just notice when it's gone off, attend to that experience for a moment, and usher your attention back gently.

There's no need to judge yourself. The mind never shuts off.

The awakening is in the noticing.

Just bring yourself back from wherever the mind went.

The breath is the way to return.

You might release the thought by simply labeling it as "thinking."

If you experience any discomfort, just notice it objectively, with equanimity. Everything you feel is perfectly natural. Allow yourself to be curious and meet what's there, whether those sensations and thoughts are pleasant or unpleasant. There's no need to chase the pleasant sensations or avoid the unpleasant ones.

Just greet each one openly, with friendly, full acceptance.

Everything that you become aware of will arise, exist, and fall away. It's all impermanent. Just know it for the moment and let it go. Let it gently fall away.

Now begin to expand the field of awareness. Bring awareness to the sounds in the room. They are happening all the time. Notice the smells in the air, the taste in your mouth, and the sensations of the body meeting the seat beneath you. Sit with awareness as you witness the constant unfolding of life around you.

Life is beautifully mysterious.

Just notice what is here to be seen.

Here we meet life as it is.

Breathe, notice, and be.

Moving from Darkness to Light through Meditation

There are times when we feel so deeply lost in our struggle it is as though we are housed in our anguish, alone. This is usually when we need to remind ourselves, "It's OK to not be OK." You might hold your burdens firm to your chest or your emotions may spill out everywhere and with everyone. These moments of pain feel so personal and permanent that we can find the body feeling locked into suffering and the mind focused so steadily on the hurt that it feels perpetual and insurmountable. In these dark times, we forget our resilience and the extraordinary capacity of the human heart to endure. But when we are willing to open to even the most unimaginable of difficulties and enter the quiet stillness of meditation, we can transform our pain into a heart wisdom that informs our life.

Meditation calls us to detach from thoughts, feelings, and bodily sensations and observe them compassionately. When we sit with them, with kindness, and anchor into awareness, we discover an inner spaciousness—space that allows deep-held *sankhara* (conditions of the mind such as memories, images, and mental or emotional patterns) to arise, exist, and dissolve. It is space that allows us to see these conditions in a new light and to let them go. This space is like an ocean of self-discovery. In time we settle into the quiet mystery below the surface of the mental and emotional storms, a vast and peaceful awareness.

Compassion Meditation

Every style of meditation is about educating the heart and mind and cultivating loving kindness. The minute we take our seat to practice, we've taken a radical act toward love. Compassion meditation is a way to enter into a deliberate and structured practice of fostering loving kindness. It acknowledges the interconnectedness of all living things and the profound impact of coordinating our heart, mind, body, and spirit. It is an intentional commitment to our own inner peace and happiness and also to the well-being of all. You'll find a beautiful Metta meditation for mothers in chapter 13 with information about how to adapt it for your daily practice (whether or not you are a parent). You'll also find the compassion practice of Tonglen in chapter 10. It's like a tonic for difficult emotions and can relieve suffering during challenging times. I encourage you to include some form of compassion meditation daily (it takes only minutes to sink into the heart center and hold the wish that others be safe, happy, healthy, and free from suffering) and it's a deeply honoring way to close your formal practice.

The Benefits of a Silent Meditation Retreat

I've practiced many approaches to meditation and I can honestly say that I have never come across a technique that so thoroughly confronts the deep roots of our inner patterns as a silent meditation retreat does. Taming the mind is like taming a wild elephant. It pulls, it complains, it fights hard as we pierce the layers of egoic illusions. In time, the buildup of egoic belief systems, emotional and mental patterns, images of trauma, loss, shame, and all other roots to our suffering are loosened and metabolized. It's the most thorough mental detox imaginable.

We've all heard accounts of people changing their lives after a silent meditation retreat. They may quit their job or move to a rural village in Europe. Less radically (and much more commonly), they simply move a little slower, observe nature a bit more, and feel more peaceful and content. Retreats can be extraordinarily beneficial for providing a supportive community with which to refine our meditation practice and get to know ourselves and life better. The deep immersive nature of retreat life gives us an accurate vision of ourselves that is both humbling and awe-inspiring. We begin to see just how ordinary and Buddha-like we truly are.

If you're in a position to take advantage of a meditation retreat, go slow and steady—it may be the most important work you ever do.

Jen's Story: Afterword

I feel overwhelmingly grateful when I think about Jen's story and the ways the practice of meditation allowed her to befriend herself. Meditation is less a practice or a technique than it is a relationship, a lifelong friend. Like all good friends, it's truthful. It doesn't dance around the difficulty: it's inherently honest.

The last thing Jen felt like doing when her mind was racing with anxious thoughts was to turn her focus inward. And yet that is the exact medicine she needed. She learned that if you let it, the open awareness of meditation can be the balm that soothes internal distress not by getting rid of it but by opening to it. Meditation isn't a way of quashing or eliminating pain; it's about welcoming all that is there. With meditation we let go of control altogether, relaxing into the moment with total compassion and honesty.

Top 3 Takeaways

1. Meditation is not mystical; it is hard science. Meditation activates key regions of the brain, building the brain mass and neurological connections that support a clear, focused mind, compassion, and many health benefits.

2. Every time we meditate, we have the potential to open a gateway to the awe and wonder of our own potential.

3. Meditation will, in time, bring ease but it's really the way to awaken to what's truly there. Expect discomfort, and welcome it as an opportunity to learn to witness the changing flow of inner experience with openness and equanimity.

Journal Prompts

- What expectations are you carrying about what meditation should provide you?

- What would help you to enter into your practice with a beginner's mind, curious and open?

- What are you willing to give up, put aside, or release in order to claim your practice?

- Life with a daily meditation practice is like removing distortion goggles. As you meditate, what is becoming clearer? In what ways is your perspective changing?

- In what ways would you like to take the learnings from your meditation practice off the mat and embody them in your everyday life?

4

Presence

Mindfulness and Equanimity

"You cannot find yourself in the past or future.
The only place where you can find yourself is in the Now."

ECKHART TOLLE

Kendra's Story

"My God, when I think about all the times that I've obsessed about what I said to a friend or worried because a colleague didn't give me the time of day, I've spent the better part of my life ruminating about things I have zero control over and whether I'm good enough in other people's eyes. I'm over it, Michele, but I have no idea how to stop. My mind just takes over altogether, and I'm just along for the ride."

Kendra has a sparky energy that I can't help delighting in. She is resilient, openhearted, and loves to have conversations about con-sciousness and karma and existential angst. She's the kind of client

I can imagine having dinner with (but obviously wouldn't). When she first came to me, she was self-aware enough to see the ways that her internal mind patterns were leading to periods of deep unhappiness and angst. "I just want to turn off my brain," she said. "Can't you teach me how to turn off my thoughts? You seem so peaceful!"

What we see in others can be deceptive. Kendra didn't have a window into my patterns of ruminating and self-judging and the many times my mind took me off into the abyss. I told her that I haven't yet found a way to turn off the thinking mind (not even while I sleep), but there are some ways to work with it to stabilize it. "When we befriend the mind and learn to observe it without adding more to the thinking, it becomes less of an obstacle," I told her. "Through the everyday practice of mindfulness, you can learn to avoid getting caught up with the thinking mind. And you can find your way toward greater compassion for yourself."

While we all struggle with rumination, our life experiences contribute to our individual mind patterns. For example, when I asked Kendra about her relationships with her family she quickly centered on her father, describing him as complex, reactive, and impossible to please. She never quite knew what would set her dad off, and when he was triggered, Kendra would endure long rants that often erupted into explosive anger. She had learned to read her father's facial expressions, body language, and emotional tone, scanning his cues to confirm whether she was in the safe or unsafe zone. As Kendra tried to understand what she had or had not done to set him off, a pattern of self-doubt developed that had endured in every relationship since. What Kendra wanted so badly was to create a friendlier, more accepting relationship with her mind. She wanted the peace and joy that are her birthright.

In this chapter we'll look at the thinking mind and the simple yet powerful ways to find peace in the present. You'll discover that with practice it's possible to shape the brain to accept life exactly as it is, even the painful parts, and move into a calmer and more consciously aware life.

Learning to Live Fully in the Present

If you closed your eyes now and became very still, what would you notice? You might become aware of the sensation of your breath or your heart beating or the tension you're holding in your shoulders. But it wouldn't take long before you started listening to that very familiar and constant inner chatter. In no time at all, the inner voice carries us into stories and judgments and narratives about ourselves and the world around us. This discursive thinking is the egoic mind. You, the true essence of you, is the listener of that egoic mind—the true essence of you is consciousness itself.

If you observed the inner voice in your head long enough, chances are it took you into thoughts of the future or the past. If you were swept away into thoughts of the future, they likely followed a story line of anticipation, worry, or fear. Future-focused fear-based thinking breeds anxiety. Your inner dialogue might sound something like this:

"My boss wants to meet with me. What if he's firing me?"

"Last time I spoke with my father it was a disaster. Tonight's dinner will just be the same."

"What if my daughter hates her new school? She'll end up blaming me forever!"

We find ourselves pulled into this kind of thinking all the time. When we get caught up in the ego's insatiable appetite for catastrophic, fear-focused, and unequivocally untrue thoughts, they can become the architecture of our personality and the basis of a lifetime of suffering.

But the inner voice doesn't limit itself to creating negative perceptions of the future. It also loves to replay our perceptions of events of the past, often in critical and regretful ways. I say "perceptions" because our memories are largely made up of fragments of narratives that become increasingly inaccurate over time. Research has shown that what we tell ourselves about a memory is the core determining factor in how we feel about the event itself.[1] You might recognize these inner dialogues:

"That last breakup was so painful. If I'd been more up-front, maybe we could have made it work."

"Why didn't I start that business concept last year? I would be in a very different place by now."

"If only I had been more present with my son, maybe he wouldn't be struggling in this way."

Replaying and beating ourselves up over events of the past becomes a loveless pattern. It is the psyche's way of grasping and holding on to the pain of the past. Why does this happen? The egoic mind becomes attached to the drama story, rerunning the internal narrative over and over again to master or change life's difficulties. It doesn't have the wisdom to know that just because something happened in the past doesn't mean it'll happen again. The ego also oversimplifies, judging the past, attaching thoughts of right or wrong, good or bad, and our emotion centers respond in kind. We're left feeling anxious and unavailable to what's right in front of us, the raw beauty of life in the present moment.

Now imagine another reality. A lived reality based on a loving and accepting relationship with your internal self, where, on a moment-to-moment basis, you open to the unfolding of your thoughts, feelings, and experiences. You do this not through the lens of the future or the past, but through the lens of present time— the only place that is true and real. Change your relationship with the mind and you will alter not only how you meet life but also your whole reality.

Imagine for a moment that in your desire to learn more about your emotional patterns (and particularly how to improve them), you stumble across an app that promises to help you track your mood and isolate which aspects of your life help bolster it. In no time at all you've downloaded the app, and within a few hours you receive your first check-in.

"*How do you feel?*" the app asks. You think to yourself, "I'm in a busy grocery store in the middle of a pandemic. How do you think I feel?" The app gives you a range of options, from Very Bad to Very

Good. You move the cursor across the scale to show you're feeling unhappy and a little agitated.

The app then wants to know, "*What are you doing?*" You scan the categories and land on the one that seems to fit closest.

The app asks a few more questions and then it goes on to the key question, "*Are you thinking about something other than what you are currently doing?*" Your neural receptors start firing as you think to yourself, "Let's see, I was picking through the bananas, internally freaking out about the man next to me who was getting way too close for comfort, but what was I actually thinking about?" And then it comes to you. "I was thinking about what might happen if I get sick and the impact that will have on my husband, and then what if he gets sick, and so on and so on." "*No,*" you type into the app, "*I was definitely not thinking about the bananas, or even the way I was maneuvering away from the man-hoverer. I was down the rabbit hole of all of the horrible things that I was certain would happen.*" You quickly answer a few more questions and move on with your errands.

That first interaction with the app reveals a seed of insight. You discover you may be tuned out to the truth of what's actually happening *most* of the time. That in fact, you're like Alice in Wonderland going down rabbit hole after rabbit hole and living in an absurd alternative universe. And that you've managed to convince yourself that you're at death's door because a man stepped slightly shy of six feet away from you.

As the weeks go on, the app randomly sends you more signals throughout the day. It pings when you're brushing your teeth, on your way to work, and while you're cooking dinner. It even pings when you're having sex. In time you begin to see patterns in the ways that your happiness rises and falls, and while the app doesn't really tell you for sure, you can sense that it seems to be guiding you toward greater self-awareness.

Wouldn't it be great if this app were real? The truth is over 15,000 people have actually used it. The human behind the app, the neurobiologist and happiness researcher Matt Killingsworth, has collected data from people in eighty countries.[2] While *they* were in the produce aisle accounting for their happiness levels, thoughts, and all kinds of other data, they were adding to the data bank of another 650,000 real-time reports.

It turns out that as you did this exercise the connections you may have been making intuitively between your feelings of happiness and your state of mind were also true for a significant number of other participants—especially when it came to the wandering mind. In fact, according to Killingsworth's study, mind-wandering is strongly correlated with unhappiness. When the app users were focused on the past or the future, they reported feeling happy only 56 percent of the time. However, when their mind was focused on the present moment, they reported feeling happy 66 percent of the time. They were significantly happier when attuned to the present moment! And it didn't matter what they were doing. Whether people were working, running errands, spending time with friends, brushing their teeth, or having sex, they were happier if they were focused on the "now."

You might be thinking to yourself, "What if my mind is focused on the past or the future but I'm dreaming about or recounting something pleasant? How can that be negative? Maybe I'm thinking about how amazing I felt when I first met my partner or the plans I'm making for my girlfriend's fortieth birthday." According to Killingsworth's discovery, mind-wandering may not offer the lift from the day-to-day we hope for. In fact, wandering around even the most pleasant of rabbit holes contributes to lower happiness levels, perhaps not as much as unpleasant past and future thoughts, but lower nonetheless.

Now remember your realization about just how often you're jumping into that mental vortex? Well, it turns out you were on to something. Your mind is focused on the moment only 47 percent of the time, at least according to Killingsworth's data. That's almost half of our life that we're missing.

If being in the moment is so important to our happiness levels, how do we then draw from the past to use our experiences in ways that inspire, empower, and guide us forward? The secret is in the return. Our perceptions of the past are like avatars, representations of how we believe things to have been. Over time these avatars shift and transform until we internalize these distorted narratives as *truth*. Instead, we can draw on perceptions of the past without losing ourselves in the narratives. The problem for Alice in Wonderland wasn't falling down the rabbit hole; it was her inability to return to her real life.

How does the future fit in? If being in the present is so important to our well-being, how can we then plan and innovate and prepare for what's to come? When we think ahead, we can begin to design and organize our life. Envisioning is a woman's superpower! It allows us to actualize our gifts and desires. The secret is to envision our aspirations clearly, to set them in motion, and then to return to the beauty of what's happening right in front of us. Reconstructing our inner life to become more present is a continual practice of shifting awareness. As you practice, you'll fall out of your intention, forget, lose awareness, find yourself living in the stories of the past or the future time and time again. But eventually you'll more easily escort your awareness back to life as it is now, with kindness and acceptance. We transcend our own illusions by opening ourselves to the moment as it is, and we begin to thrive in the spaciousness of present time.

Arriving into Present Time

TIME NEEDED: 13 MINUTES

THIS MEDITATION TEACHES us to find refuge in the present moment. We'll trace the paths between the past, the future, and the now, teaching the mind how to intentionally find its way back to the spaciousness of this moment.

Turn inward by closing your eyes or rest the gaze slightly down and in front of you. Feel the body where it makes contact with the support beneath you and allow yourself to settle into the moment.

Breathe through the nose.

Feel the breath as it enters the body, and with each exhale begin to let go of any tension. Or bring attention to the sensation of the breath at the belly if that's easier for you.

Noticing now the natural inhale and natural exhale.

There is nowhere else to go and no better thing to do than this. Simply be in the awareness of the breath. Thoughts will arise. Emotions and sensations will arise. Just notice them for the moment and let them be. Let them go. Allow them to pass through the mind like a leaf on a stream or bubbles on the Ganges River. You might label them as "thinking" as they float on by. Return to the breath each time the mind wanders.

Noticing the sensation of the incoming breath and the outgoing breath.

Awakening to life as it is right here, right now. Be aware of the sounds in the room, the smells in the air, the taste in your mouth, and the sensations of the body as you sit.

Resting in the unending now.

Now bring to your awareness an event from the past—nothing too painful or difficult though. It may be something that happened recently or years ago. Picture that event clearly and feel it deeply. Notice the reaction in the thinking mind. Notice the emotions that emerge and any changes in the body, meeting whatever arises with openness and kindness.

Bring your awareness back to the breath.

Return to your awareness of this moment where the past is no more. Again, be aware of the sounds in the room, the smells in the air, the taste in your mouth, and the sensations of the body.

Now focus your attention on a future event. It may be something that you have planned for later this evening, tomorrow, or even years from now. Whatever it is, however you see it, visualize it clearly and feel it deeply. Notice the reaction in the thinking mind. Notice the emotions that emerge and the reaction in the body.

Again, let that go, anchor in the breath, anchor in the now. Attune to the sounds, the smells in the air, the taste in your mouth, and the sensations of the body as you sit in quiet stillness, right here, right now.

Breathe, notice, and be.

Gently open your eyes. Place your hand on your heart and set the intention to walk through your day resting in the gift of the unending now, deeply, compassionately, present to whatever may arise in each moment.

Locus of Control

While training the mind to be in the present is a big part of fostering inner steadiness, the mind has many other habits that can interfere with our ability to be present and open to experiencing the joy that's right in front of us. Have you noticed how often the mind focuses (if not obsesses) on the external? We all experience this tendency to some degree. We look to find happiness in a better job, a new partner, or other changes outside ourselves that we've been told will grant us joy. Or we convince ourselves that if we were more accomplished, thinner, more educated, or affluent, our worries and anxieties might disappear. The idea that more is better is very seductive in our culture. We grasp for the next thing, and the next thing after that, anxiously seeking to affirm our sense of self. And while some of those factors may bring temporary happiness and should be enjoyed, a part of us recognizes that they will not bring enduring peacefulness. Why is this so? Because each of us is already whole.

We've all met people who are deeply happy with very little. And yet many people with a lot are deeply unhappy. Why is this pattern of overfocusing on external things so difficult to resist? One of my all-time favorite research studies reveals some astounding cultural trends and the impact they have on our worldview. Jean Twenge, a professor of psychology at San Diego State University, conducted two major studies examining locus of control, or the degree to which people believe their lives are controlled by internal versus external forces.[3] One study showed "the average college student in 2002 had a more external locus of control than 80% of college students in the early 1960s."[4] The study also highlights that looking outside of ourselves for a sense of worth or for answers to finding enduring happiness is almost uniformly negative. An externally focused life is associated with helplessness, greater difficulty managing stress, lower academic achievement, feelings of loss of control, and depression. According to Twenge, we are more individualistic, cynical, and self-serving than we once were (that's not great news).

But here comes the good news. If, however, we learn to adjust our internal compass with everyday practices that honor our positive internal qualities, we have the capacity to change not only our sense of well-being but also the entire direction of our life. Our mind-set and the cultural values we're taught to orient our lives toward deeply influence whether we look for happiness outside ourselves or open our hearts and minds to the happiness already within us.

Thankfully humanity has a way of autocorrecting when we veer off track. We don't need to look far to see how we are being asked to challenge and deconstruct these limiting patterns.[5] These are wisdom adjustments, moments of integrating greater awareness. They are a collective invitation toward radical healing and consciousness-raising.

The Ripple Effect

Just over a decade ago, I formally committed to Buddhism, a step known as taking refuge. I had been Buddhism-curious since the age of sixteen, studying under various Buddhist teachers and doing my best to follow the Eightfold Path of Buddhist practices. The teachings of interconnectedness, warmheartedness, and the values of the Eightfold Path resonated deeply with me. So when I was offered the chance to take refuge under Tai Situ Rinpoche, considered a living Buddha under Tibetan Buddhist tradition, I felt deeply fortunate. One of the main points of taking refuge is to acknowledge we are truly groundless, releasing ourselves from the need for security. Instead, we commit to being self-reliant and to working on ourselves with radical self-honesty.

Tai Situ Rinpoche cut my hair as a symbol of turning away from the distractions of ordinary life, placed water on my head as a gesture of purification, and gave me my dharma name, Karma Rigzen Lhamo. A dharma name reflects the tradition and lineage of the teacher and the intention of letting go of the old self. When taking refuge, we're asked to examine ourselves with full honesty and use our own inner resources and contemplative practice to guide us as we pull up our own socks, so to speak. In so doing, we begin to discover our own Buddha nature.

I often hear women say, "I know I should prioritize self-care but how on earth can I fit it into my life?" It's a legitimate question! The practices that can leave us feeling better and even extend our life often become just another thing that we "should" be doing in an already very busy life. Imagine instead turning these "shoulds" into desires. Getting to know and expressing our core desires empowers us toward full agency. For example, saying "I truly want to meditate every morning" feels different than "I really should fit meditation into my day." So begin to ask, "What do I truly want for myself?" and let those core desires lead you into a lifetime of embodied self-care.

The idea is to *use* the mind to strengthen the positive qualities that already lie within us. As we do, we begin to free ourselves from the egoic mind and all its fears, criticisms, and restrictions. With focused effort and practice using meditation and other contemplative techniques, we can begin to strengthen the parts of the brain that cultivate equanimity, self-compassion, empathy, the ability to feel fully and regulate emotion. Happiness begins to flourish naturally[6]—and the attachment to the external dissolves. Situ Rinpoche has said, "Every sentient being is equal to the Buddha." By developing our own path of awareness, compassion, and inner wisdom, we are also better able to help other people. This is the ripple effect.

Shaping the Brain for Greater Well-Being

The mind's main priority is our survival, not our happiness. But thoughts are not the enemy. Just like the body, the mind can be shaped in empowering ways. The conditioned mind can be reinforced for stronger pathways of agitation, judgment, and rigidity, or reshaped for calm and open awareness. Imagine the possibilities if we were to provide the mind with clear teachings so that it could serve us better. Keep in mind the brain has a negativity bias— it remembers punishment over praise—that can lead us to believe that the world is an unfriendly place. This negativity bias helped our ancestors survive by priming us to be vigilant about danger, but with practice and the process of neuroplasticity (more on this below) the brain will begin to interrupt harmful feedback loops and reshape pathways. We become less fearful of imagined dangers and begin to trust in our inherent safety.

With the help of advances in neuroscience, long gone are the days when we could say you can't teach an old dog new tricks. With practices that cultivate greater self-awareness, we see the inspiring potential for personal transformation.[7] As we deconstruct old fears, disentangle from patterns of hurt and reactivity, and soothe our pain points, the brain reshapes. Neuroplasticity is the brain's ability to change in size and shape and to reorganize synaptic connections. Stress has a bidirectional impact on neuroplasticity. Long-term exposure to the stress hormone cortisol alters the brain's plasticity (especially in areas related to perceived danger when there is none) in ways that make us more anxious and less able to pay attention and stay focused. Under different conditions, neuroplasticity also helps the brain to restructure in ways that foster resilience.[8]

Mindfulness practices in particular have been found to create functional neuroplastic changes in key regions of the brain associated with the stress response.[9] With as little as three days of meditation training, activity in the amygdala (the part of the brain associated with the fight-or-flight response) has been shown to decrease while connections between the mid-prefrontal cortex (the logical thinking hemisphere of the brain) and the amygdala increase. In other words, mindfulness has been found to strengthen the neural connections in key areas that mitigate the effects of stress, cultivate compassion for others,[10] and improve our ability to remain present and focused.[11] And if recent scientific claims are correct, learning and integrating mindfulness may just be the path to freeing the mind from the pain of constantly ruminating about life by dampening activity in regions of the brain associated with symptoms of suffering such as craving, aversion, and a lack of equanimity.[12]

Equanimity: Becoming Steady in the Mindstorm

For me, one of the most poignant descriptions of equanimity is written by Buddhist author Toni Bernhard: "Every moment of equanimity is waking up from the delusion that things should be as we want them to be." Equanimity is the ability to remain steady and balanced in a sustained way, especially in the face of discomfort. With equanimity we can be with the movement of the mind, allowing pain and comfort to exist at the same time.

For over a decade I trained almost exclusively in the dharma (teachings) of the Buddha, committing my evenings and weekends to long retreats and contemplative practice. It was like Buddha boot camp for developing equanimity. While my practice looks a little gentler now (I've found my middle path), I'm grateful for the discipline it taught me. Facing ourselves with full honesty requires a committed effort in a world that worships the external. And yet when we dedicate ourselves to the practice of inner reflection, we begin to starkly see the patterns that trip us up and keep us mired in suffering. We discover a life liberated from negative stories, judgments, and reactivity. We learn to see reality as it is, pleasant and unpleasant—not from a place of indifference, but with a clear and equanimous mind.

According to the Buddha, the commonality for us all is the unavoidable experience of suffering. In other words, it's really hard to be a person sometimes. Things just keep happening to us, and the mind inevitably gets involved. In our natural tendency to prevent pain, the mind begins to work hard to protect us, turning away in aversion rather than staying with what's occurring. So when we go through something stressful, we argue against it, telling ourselves that it shouldn't be so, adding layers of resentment, fear, and other painful emotions. When instead we face these stressors with a sense of equanimity, or nonreaction, we become more open to life as it's happening. With equanimity we can experience life more fully, enlivened rather than taken down emotionally by the difficulties. This doesn't mean that we become inactive or allow ourselves to be pushed around—quite the opposite. In experiencing life fully and openly, we can respond to challenges more thoughtfully. An equanimous mind is clear and awake, the precise condition that relieves the discomfort we were so trying to avoid in the first place.

If we take a moment to think about the many textures of emotion that run through us, it's no wonder that we sometimes feel overwhelmed. And while our emotions are layered and nuanced with information, it can be difficult to discern what they are and what they mean. According to researchers from New York University, human beings experience up to twenty-seven emotions.[13] That's a whole lot of feeling going on! Those emotional experiences can range from extremely pleasant (the pleasures of sex or chocolate, or the wonder of birth) to unimaginably unpleasant (the loss of a loved one or the pain from a serious injury). Life is a steady stream of emotional and cognitive experiences, all impermanent.

Consider a typical day. You wake up to the sight of your partner bringing you coffee: pleasant. Then you use the toilet and discover you're out of toilet paper: unpleasant. You open your yoga mat and start the day with asanas: pleasant. You lose track of time and rush to work: unpleasant. You arrive late and your boss gives you a stern look: unpleasant. A coworker invites you to lunch at a new café down the street: pleasant. You can see the pattern of ups and downs. We push the unpleasant moments away and long for pleasant ones to arrive. We find ourselves caught in a constant cycle of craving and aversion, wishing for more pleasure and turning away from pain.

Imagine training the mind to stay where you are. How might your life be different if you could face the joys and sorrows without labeling them as good or bad, right or wrong? Our reality is but one perspective of life. It is like a fun mirror that reflects everything we see, yet shaped and distorted by our perceptions and internal conditions. Everything in our path can teach us and wake us up to life's full scope, but it takes time and practice looking at that mirror with a kinder perspective to show the mind a way toward the peace and freedom of equanimity.

MEDITATION

Training the Mind for Equanimity

TIME NEEDED: 14 MINUTES

THIS MEDITATION WILL strengthen your ability to welcome both the pleasant and unpleasant aspects to life with equanimity and openheartedness. You'll need a timer for this exercise. Set the alarm to ring gently at the end of each minute, for nine minutes.

Turn inward by closing your eyes.

And begin to notice the sensation of the breath.

The breath entering the body and the breath leaving the body.

You might notice yourself being soothed by the incoming and outgoing breath.

Notice where you can connect with the breath naturally. Maybe it's the sensation of the breath at the nostril, or above the upper lip, or you might feel its wave swell at the belly or as it ripples through the body. See what feels most natural for you.

Let the heart be tender and open to receive whatever arises with acceptance.

Now allow the mind to intentionally bring forward any unpleasant thoughts you've been carrying. Welcome and usher in the thoughts you normally avoid and push away. It may feel counterintuitive, but call in the thoughts of worry and fear and resentment. Willingly spend a little time with the uncomfortable thoughts. Allow them all. Now begin to observe those thoughts with a friendliness and a sense of curiosity and compassion. Notice what happens when you do. You might see that they shift and change in this environment of kindness. See if you can witness the thoughts with a warmheartedness. Remember, they're just thoughts. Every thought is impermanent; it arises, exists, and falls away.

Now allow those unpleasant thoughts to dissolve into dust, free to dance with the wind. Call in now the many pleasant thoughts that move through the mind. Bring forward the joyful thoughts and memories. Give the pleasant thoughts your fullest attention. Notice how these thoughts also arise, exist, and fall away. They too are impermanent. Can you observe these thoughts without reacting or trying to hold on to them in the mind?

Now bring yourself back from the dream and allow those pleasant thoughts to dissolve into dust once again. Anchor in the breath, noticing what meets your awareness now. Rest in the truth of this moment, aware of the sensation of each life-affirming breath. Give full awareness to life, just as it is and without any need for it to be different. Be right here, right now. Notice the sounds in the room, the shadows behind the eyes, the taste in your mouth, and the scent as it dances through the chambers of the nose. Feel the solidity of the chair below you and the air as it grazes across the skin. Whether the sensations are pleasant or unpleasant, begin to welcome them with great tenderness. Notice too what happens in the thinking mind as you allow yourself to meet the moment, anchoring in the breath, sitting in the nowness.

Take some time now to repeat this cycle, moving from pleasant thoughts to unpleasant thoughts, to the spaciousness that comes with anchoring in present time. Spend a minute or so with each one.

Breathe, notice, and be.

At the end of this meditation, take a moment to write down anything you noticed. Maybe you noticed it was challenging to come back from the pleasant thoughts. Or perhaps you felt an aversion to the unpleasant thoughts. Did your respiration change? What emotions came forward? How about the sensations in the body? If you found this exercise difficult, try not to be hard on yourself. In time and with practice the mind learns to self-correct, escorting itself back to the now more easily.

Kendra's Story: Afterword

Kendra's process of self-healing was as much an exercise in understanding the nature of consciousness as it was in healing the emotional impact of family relationships. She was an eager student of life, enlivened by the perspective that her true self, her essence, resides in a vast field of awareness beyond the thinking mind, the body, and the personality she had worn for her entire life. She began to pause more often to interrupt the fear stories, practiced calm and open awareness through meditation, and checked in on the quality of her thinking mind throughout the day. She no longer wished she could shut off the thinking mind and discovered ways to drop under it, observing it from a greater distance. She learned to use the breath to sink into the inner calm, beneath those unending waves of thought. And perhaps the most empowering outcome for Kendra was a newfound perspective that she didn't need to act on them—especially when they were telling her she needed to make others happy to be safe in the world.

Top 3 Takeaways

1. We live in our highest well-being when we bring our fullest awareness to the present moment.

2. Our Western culture's tendency toward an externally focused life is quashing our well-being. By honoring and cultivating our internal qualities, we have access to a more enduring happiness.

3. With focused effort and practice using meditation and other contemplative techniques, we can strengthen the parts of the brain that cultivate equanimity, compassion, self-acceptance, clarity, and altruism; regulate emotion; and downplay the negativity bias.

Journal Prompts

- Do you find yourself wishing for life to be different or believing that you'll be happy when you achieve an external goal? Write about your mind habits and the ways you chase happiness outside yourself.

- Describe the ways you can shape the mind toward greater equanimity, especially in difficult times. What would you like to do or tell yourself in order to meet the moment with greater compassion?

- Notice where and when your mind wanders most often and when you feel most present. Write about the times when you get lost in the past and future and what you can do to bring yourself back to the moment.

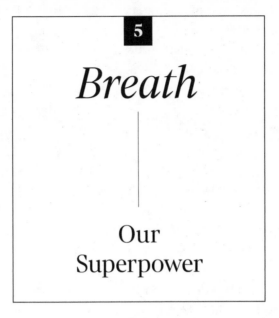

Breath

Our Superpower

"Breath is the bridge which connects life to consciousness, which unites your body to your thoughts. Whenever your mind becomes scattered, use your breath as the means to take hold of your mind again."

THICH NHAT HANH

Lori's Story

"How long do you think it'll take before I'm back to normal?" Lori asked. It's a question almost every client asks when they're facing the inordinate discomfort of anxiety. Lori had big plans for her life, and the panic attacks she'd been experiencing were not fitting well with her timelines. As with most things, she wanted an end result, even if that meant driving herself out of the moment to get there. But there's an old Zen saying that you can't push the river. Healing a burdened body takes time. Wading through painful patterns that have run deep for years, if not decades, is not an overnight process.

Lori's relationship with herself had become harsh and unforgiving: she was terribly impatient, always striving toward bigger, better, faster. Lori was consumed with her work as a lawyer and endured a schedule that seemed to be constantly accelerating. Her husband too was a lawyer. Although they wanted to have children, Lori made it very clear that she felt she had to establish herself professionally before she would consider having a child: "I'm thirty-six years old. Most of my friends have started having kids already and I'm not even close. Sometimes I wonder if it's even in the cards. I have this biological clock that's forcing a decision and I don't want to lose out on opportunities because I decide to have a baby."

As Lori talked about her inner struggle, her breathing became shallower. I felt a tightening in my own chest as her tone and cadence quickened. I gently pointed out to Lori the shift in her body and breathing and suggested a few long exhales to soothe the nervous system. But to pause, even in therapy, felt threatening. She continued to explain that pulling back even a little just wasn't going to be possible. I explained the neuroscience behind the practice of deep breathing and the ways that it could help address her struggles with inattention, support her compromised immune system, and most importantly help quell the messages of distress and the fight-or-flight response that was causing the panic attacks. She opened a little to the possibility of doing regulated breathing exercises throughout the day.

To cope in a masculine-driven system, we often begin to match its rigidity. We become preoccupied with lists and goals and timelines and we begin to develop an "expert mind" that shuts down possibility, curiosity, and an openness to learning what life is truly showing us. For Lori, any suggestion of slowing down or listening to her body or an inner voice, or pausing to better see where she was getting caught, felt like a confrontation. She was fully committed to the ego-identity she had formed and was holding on to it tightly, defending herself against anything that looked too "soft." Nothing, especially panic attacks, could get in the way of achieving right alongside her husband.

Lori took out her phone, opened the notes section to document her plan, and we formulated some ways to better cope with the panic attacks. She agreed to try some regulated breathing a few times per day, shifting her thoughts to a more supportive inner dialogue (focusing on what was going well over what wasn't); eat more regularly; cut out coffee; and work on getting a little more sleep (she was down to six hours per night). Lori expressed a sense of relief as she left. She'd formulated the plan that she felt she needed. And while I would have loved to have helped her discover and confront the inner story that somehow she needed to prove her worth, I recognized that I too was learning gentle patience. Her path could not be shaped in ways she wasn't ready for. For now, I knew each breath would support her faithfully.

Healing through Conscious Breath

Breath is life. This we know. She doesn't move through us; she is us, invisible and essential. Breath is energy and consciousness itself. Her healing current is the medicine that vibrates through every cell of our being. She carries oxygen to our blood, lungs, and heart, purifying as she traces the path to the places most in need. She feeds the cells of our tissues and organs and then carries away and expels the toxins and pollutants. She affirms our life, sustains us faithfully, and releases us from the body when it's time. When we partner with her, the capacity for healing and well-being swells like a flower painted by Georgia O'Keeffe. Supported, she can empower the immune system, help heal from illness, extend life, and soothe what needs to be soothed.

We take an average of 20,000 breaths a day. That's 20,000 invitations to activate the healing vibration of our life-force energy and to root ourselves in the present. We know that slow, deep breathing—conscious breathing—supports health by turning up the soothing parasympathetic nervous system and tamping down the activating sympathetic nervous system, a sure route to a calmer life.[1] The vagus nerve (see page 17) plays a pivotal role in this process, communicating messages to the brain to set off the relaxation response. The breathing exercises you'll find in this chapter are vagal maneuvers that slow down the heart rate and set off a cascade of healing responses. The breath is undoubtedly one of the most potent antidotes to stress and a key part of any practice.

Take a moment now and draw in a low and slow conscious breath, pause, and radiate an even longer exhale. Breathe through the nose. Inhale for a count of four, pause for four, and exhale completely for a count of six. Now hold for two. Keep following that breath pattern (4, 4, 6, 2) a few more times. What do you notice? A relaxing of the muscles? A slowing down of the heart? A moment between thoughts? A sense of your own presence? Greater awareness? Do you feel greater ease, if even for a moment?

Conscious breathing is a mechanism for healing. It allows us to get calm enough, long enough to see what life is showing us. The relaxed breath soothes our inner agitation, anxiety, and panic. It dissolves mental and physical tension, and in times of fear the breath anchors us in the body. As the body calms, we can begin to listen to our emotions with wisdom and awareness. The breath shows us the way to let go and open to what's there, to metabolize our fears naturally. A single breath can return us to the moment and make us more fully available to both the pleasant and unpleasant parts of life all at the same time. The calming effect can also open portals to consciousness we may not have visited before, to the space between our thoughts where awareness lies.

Our breath is the most powerful tool we have to self-soothe. The trick is to breathe slowly and deeply at nonanxious times to avoid getting into those sticky states in the first place. As we focus on the breath, a shift takes place inside us, an irreversible awakening process, where we transcend thought and emotion to touch the expansiveness of our true nature.

Resetting the Breath

Depending on the quality of the breath, we can meet each moment with suppression, radiance, or anything in between. The breath supports a reserve of energy that not only absorbs oxygen and expels carbon dioxide, but also eliminates the buildup of toxins that cause illness.[2]

As we face strong negative emotions, the fight-or-flight response unconsciously activates the respiratory center of the brain, speeding up the breath. The breath becomes shallow and the air moves clumsily through the upper chambers of the lungs rather than the lower diaphragm, which disrupts the balance of gases in the body.

Fortunately, we also have the capacity to partner with the breath in ways that can optimize the respiratory system and transform our well-being. To ignore the breath is to close down one of the most powerful portals to health. With each deep breath we naturally align our heart rate with our breathing. This synchronicity leads the brain to release endorphins, neurochemicals that have a naturally calming effect. Imagine, even the simplest shift in breathing can recalibrate the chemical balance in the body and draw in a natural medicine that serves us in more challenging times. So while we may not be able to singlehandedly shut down the burning of fossil fuels, the genetically modified organisms in our food, and the injustices of oppression, we *can* choose to use our breath to live healthier and more consciously.

The breath is chronically undervalued as a healing tool in the Western medical canon, but our ancestors recognized its power and value. Did you know that they gently pinched their babies' mouths closed after feeding to encourage nose breathing? They understood that teaching their children to breathe "low and slow" through the nose, rather than the mouth, would amplify a sense of inner calm and improve many aspects of mind-body health and development.[3]

I've heard from countless women about the ways in which breath training has fortified them and expanded their well-being. And whether I'm teaching breath workshops to executives, new moms, or to wellness conference-goers, I'm told the same thing: I had no idea how important my breath is. Women who arrived feeling fragile and out of control have described feeling remarkably calmer, clear minded, and connected to themselves again. In more dramatic cases, students have described being freed from their body into other planes of consciousness or having flown with God. The multidimensional space around us is usually well beyond our conscious awareness, but breath work seems to untether the egoic mind and give us more open access to consciousness itself.

Every now and again a scientific study comes along that turns our previous outlook on its head. The Framingham Study, which was started more than seventy years ago by the Boston Medical Center, is one of those studies.[4] The scientific team has followed four generations of 5,000-plus participants and continues to do so today. As far as research goes, this study is outstanding in its scope and duration. Although it was initiated to better understand family patterns of heart disease, the data and genetic information allowed researchers to discover so much more than they had hoped for. Most significantly, they found that the most accurate marker of health and longevity was not genetics or heart health as had long been presumed but lung capacity and respiratory health. In other words, the quality of a person's breathing matters most. Along with several other key findings, the data from this study support what Buddhists and yoga practitioners have been suggesting for thousands of years: the ideal breath rate for a long and healthy life seems to be five breaths per minute.

Just a few minutes a day is all you need to reset your breathing. The beautiful thing is breath work is a form of self-care that can slide easily into your day. Practice whenever and wherever is convenient for you.

Zazen Counting Breath

TIME NEEDED: 3 MINUTES

ZAZEN IS A simple Zen Buddhist practice to retrain breathing patterns and cultivate an open, calm, and stable mind.

1. Find a comfortable and secure place to sit, either cross-legged on the floor or on a firm chair. Slightly bow the chin. Lengthen the spine and bring the body forward, away from the back of the chair.

2. Rest the hands in one another, palms facing up, thumbs gently touching. Rest the gaze on the ground a few feet in front of you, eyes partially closed.

3. Breathe through the nose and rest the tongue lightly against the upper palate.

4. Let the breath be deep, restful, effortless. Body, breath, mind: inseparable. Give the breath your fullest attention.

5. Now count as you exhale, 1, 2, 3, 4, 5. And count as you inhale, 1, 2, 3, 4, 5.

6. Count with each breath and open to the sensation as the belly gently rises and falls.

   When a thought arises and you lose yourself in it, just bring your attention back to the counting.

7. Counting as you exhale, 1, 2, 3, 4, 5. Counting as you inhale, 1, 2, 3, 4, 5.

   Breathe, notice, and be.

The Perils of Mouth Breathing

You'll notice that the breathing exercises throughout this book encourage you to breathe through the nose. An estimated 25 to 50 percent of us are chronic mouth breathers.[5] But when we gulp air in and out through the mouth, whether by daytime habit or snoring and mouth breathing at night, we interfere with the body's optimal exchange of oxygen and carbon dioxide.

The nose warms the air we breathe and creates the conditions for better absorption of the air by the lungs. Its tiny little hairs, called cilia, are thought to filter out over 20 billion particles each day. Nose breathing oxygenates the lower lungs, which are rich with nerve receptors that support the parasympathetic nervous system. Chest and mouth breathing, in contrast, lead the air right to the sympathetic nerve receptors which turn on the fight-or-flight response.

This next exercise will strengthen your nose breathing ability, slow your breathing rhythm, and drive oxygen into the lower lungs to fill your cup with calm. It's one of my favorite breathing exercises, a wonderful tool to smooth out the emotional edges before a meeting or to hone the resonance in the body before formal meditation.

Nadi Shodhana
(Alternate Nostril Breathing)

TIME NEEDED: 4 MINUTES

WITH NADI SHODHANA (also known as alternate nostril breathing), you'll use the flow of the breath to clear the mind and calm the nervous system. *Nadi* means "flow" and *shodhana* means "purification." This simple practice quickly decreases the stress response, driving air into the lower area of the lungs, improving oxygen levels, and filtering pathogens to prevent disease. It activates the parasympathetic nervous system through the vagus nerve.

I first learned Nadi Shodhana from Shari, a wisdom teacher in Northern India who had learned the technique decades earlier from her guru. Later she traveled to Canada and became an unwavering voice for the dharma of compassion, unity, and service. She pushed against gender bias and resistance from both male and female members of her temple. But in time her clarity and pure heart magnetized the teachings, and students came from all over the world to learn. "If you do breath exercises every day, you will never die," she told me. Shari's radiance was enough to convince me. "I've been practicing this yogic technique for over thirty years and I never get sick. It will give you a long, healthy life."

1. Find a comfortable sitting position cross-legged on the floor or upright in a chair. Lengthen the spine and open at the heart.

2. Relax your left palm comfortably into your lap. Bring your right hand just in front of your face.

3. Bring the pointer finger and middle finger to rest between the eyebrows, lightly use them as an anchor. The fingers you'll actively use are the thumb and ring finger.

4. Close your eyes and take a deep breath in and out through the nose.

5. Close the right nostril with the right thumb. Inhale through the left nostril slowly and steadily.

6. Close the left nostril with your ring finger so both nostrils are held closed.

7. Open the right nostril and release the breath slowly through the right side. Pause briefly at the bottom of the exhale.

8. Inhale through the right side slowly.

9. Hold both nostrils closed (with ring finger and thumb).

10. Open the left nostril and release the breath slowly through the left side. Pause briefly at the bottom of the exhale.

11. Inhale through the left side slowly.

12. Continue alternating between each nostril slowly.

Breathe, notice, and be.

Sudarshan Kriya
(Purifying and Unblocking)

TIME NEEDED: 2 MINUTES

SUDARSHAN IS A Sanskrit word meaning "proper vision," and *kriya* means "to purify the body." Sudarshan Kriya is a yogic science that purifies the body by expanding the diaphragm muscle, elevating oxygen levels, and clearing out toxins. It's a beautiful way to start or end your day. Within minutes of beginning the practice, your heartbeat slows, your blood pressure lowers, and your fight-or-flight response becomes disarmed: the body begins to trust that it is safe. Science has supported its value with over seventy independent studies reporting its benefits to mind-body health:

- One week of daily practice = 21% increase in reported life satisfaction

- Two weeks of daily practice = 56% reduction in cortisol

- Four weeks of daily practice = 23% reduction in nonclinical anxiety, 73% reduction in clinical anxiety and 41% reported remission, and 63% reduction in nonclinical everyday blues.[6]

The practice of Sudarshan Kriya is beautifully structured to direct the current of the breath, inflating the lungs and expanding lung capacity. When you change the position of the arms, you direct the airflow to expand the diaphragm's range of motion. This expansion minimizes the dead space, or volume of air in each breath that doesn't participate in the exchange of oxygen to carbon dioxide. The full and open breaths of Sudarshan Kriya help nourish the lower part of the lungs with oxygenated air, to soothe the nervous system and the anxious mind.

But Sudarshan Kriya is so much more than a breathing exercise. When paired with positive emotion, it can unblock held trauma, strengthen psychophysiological coherence (when the physical body is harmonized by positive emotional states), and help rebuild a sense of safety within the body.

To work with this potential more fully, take a moment to connect with the intuitive wisdom that guides your ability to self-heal. Bring awareness to the sensations of the body, scanning from the top of the head down to the soles of the feet and ask yourself, What do I most need in this moment? Am I calling in a sense of calm, grace, or ease? Or does my heart long for something else altogether?

And then begin to ask, What am I ready to release? Am I freeing myself from tension, fear, or agitation or perhaps from another emotion that isn't serving me? And finally, before you begin, check in with the heart center and inquire, Am I willing to compassionately open myself to all that is arising and moving through?

Let's begin.

1. Start by kneeling on the floor, resting your weight on the legs to avoid placing stress on the knees (Vajrasana pose), or sit in any other position that allows the spine to be long. Close your eyes, relax the jaw, and soften the belly.

2. Breathe through the nose. Inhale slowly for eight counts, pause at the top of the breath, exhale slowly for eight counts. As you regulate the breath, focus on breathing low and slow. Inhale that which you most need and exhale that which is ready to release.

3. Place the hands on the hips, keeping the elbows firm and the heart soft. This position expands the base of the lungs. Breathe in slowly for four counts. Hold the breath for four. Exhale slowly for six counts. Hold for two. Repeat this cycle for ten rounds.

4. Place your hands comfortably in your lap. Breathe naturally, and as you do, scan your awareness. Notice the sensation in the body and the energetic current moving through. Inhale that which you most need and exhale that which is ready to release.

5. Place the arms in front of the chest with the thumbs under the armpits and the pointing and middle fingers touching at the heart center. This position expands the middle lungs. Breathe in slowly for four counts. Hold the breath for four. Exhale slowly for six counts. Hold for two. Repeat this cycle for ten rounds.

6. Place your hands comfortably in your lap. Breathe naturally, and as you do, scan your awareness. Notice the sensation in the body and the energetic current moving through. Inhale that which you most need and exhale that which is ready to release.

7. Bring the arms up and reach behind you until the palms of the hands reach the back of the shoulder blades. Spread the fingers apart and place the inside of the arms to the ears. This position will expand the back and top of the lungs. Breathe in slowly for four counts. Hold the breath for four. Exhale slowly for six counts. Hold for two. Repeat this cycle for ten rounds.

8. Place your hands comfortably in your lap. Breathe naturally, and as you do, scan your awareness. Notice the sensation in the body and the energetic current moving through. Inhale that which you most need and exhale that which is ready to release.

Breathe, notice, and be.

Reconstructing our inner life is a daily practice. At first, choose one breathing technique that works best for you and practice whenever is easiest. If the morning is best, choose the morning. If it's better while you wait in the car for your child to come out of school, choose that time. You'll fall out of your intention, forget, lose awareness, and find yourself out of practice over and over again. But living more gently means accepting ourselves. We transcend fear and build new habits only through unwavering self-acceptance. Simply bring yourself back to your practice and know that you are not alone. All of us are one beating heart.

Lori's Story: Afterword

It was years before I heard from Lori again. When I saw her name on my client list for the day, I was surprised and more than a little curious. Her panic attacks had subsided with the help of her previously formulated plan and even gone away completely for a while, but they were back with a vengeance. "You were such a big help when I saw you last, but I don't think I was really ready to do the work. It was such an impossibly stressful time in my career and I just didn't have the emotional room." She explained that she had been doing the breathing exercises religiously and she believed that they stopped her panic in its tracks. But no amount of breath work could counteract the pace of her life and the emotional toll of constantly trying to prove herself to herself. She wanted a gentler way. And so with her breath as her anchor she entered into a process of deep inner work that would help her to dissolve the need to prove and validate her worth. She began to see past her own identities and discovered the ways of radical self-acceptance.

Top 3 Takeaways

1. The breath is the space between our thoughts. It is pure consciousness, the place where emotions are quelled and balance is restored.

2. Each deep breath naturally aligns our heart rate with our breathing. This synchronicity leads the brain to release endorphins, chemicals that have a naturally calming effect. From this place of calm awareness, we can awaken to our lives.

3. When supported, breath helps empower the immune system, heal certain illnesses, and extend life.

Journal Prompts

- Take a few moments to observe now the sensation and cadence of your breath. Are you breathing smoothly, mindfully, through the nose? Or is the breathing shallow and rapid? Write about what the breath is telling you in this moment.

- Give light attention to your breath, slowly extending the exhale. Let the body respond, relax, and receive. What emotions are coming forward as you attune to the breath?

- How might your life be different if you gave more attention to your breath throughout the day?

- What times in the day can you naturally hitch a moment of breath awareness to (e.g., while driving, before working out or meditating, at the end of the day in bed)?

	6

Song and Mantra

The Healing Potential of Sound

*"Mantras are passwords that transform
the mundane into the sacred."*

DEVA PREMAL

Salima's Story

We often talk about the ways that chronic stress impacts our health, appetite, ability to sleep, and overall peace of mind, but rarely do we identify the ways in which it affects our auditory system. This impact hadn't occurred to me until I worked with Salima. She had muscled her way through her GMAT exams, volunteered at a local nonprofit, and studied around the clock to achieve the grades necessary to be admitted into her highly competitive MBA program. Before she had even started her first semester, she was exhausted and on the brink of burnout.

I was meeting with Salima in my office, where my therapy dog, Lloyd, had just been given a bone to maw on after several hours of patiently tending to clients. Almost as soon as Salima sat down, she straightened up in her chair and asked if Lloyd could eat his treat elsewhere. She explained, "I just can't stand the sound of chewing." I found Lloyd a comfortable spot in another room, and Salima shared more. She revealed she was the first in her family to go to university and felt pressure to succeed. She talked about how the male students in her program either overtly sabotaged her during presentations or sexually harassed her, and how the administrators of the program overlooked these actions. She also shared that as the anxiety heightened, she startled more easily and had become overly sensitive to sound. The tapping of her roommate's fingers on a computer keyboard, the crunching of an apple—any disruptions of silence led to a rush of negative emotion. Salima's cumulative stress meant her nervous system was on constant high alert for danger, and even everyday sounds left her jumpy and agitated.

Like most things that feel unbearably uncomfortable, sound was Salima's perfect teacher. We worked together to deconstruct the impact of trying to compete in a male-governed industry, and Salima talked openly about her fear of repercussions if she pushed back against her peers and professors for the daily microaggressions she faced. She was insightful and brave and armed with an arsenal of stress-reduction skills, and yet she was plagued with fear. And so we turned to sound as a pathway to healing and strengthening.

Sound is a universal and unifying part of human consciousness. Through music, sound helps us to celebrate, grieve, raise our spirits, ease a broken heart. It helps us to bond and marks the most important events of our lives. Sound can transport us back to a childhood memory, rouse us in the face of a challenge, and expand our consciousness in profound ways. It is encoded in our hearts and minds, an invisible ally to healing and transformation.

We naturally turn to sound in times of stress. Not the constant buzzing of technology or the sound of traffic, but the gentle patter of rain, the lapping of waves against the shoreline, the singing of birds, or the voice of a loved one can all soothe an anxious heart and mind. But sound is so much more than what we experience with our ears. Sound vibration resonates through our entire body and connects us to a bigger whole. When we pair mindfulness with deep listening, we open to life's fullness where the jarring sound of drilling and the melody of birds chirping (and everything in between) can live in our awareness harmoniously.

From a Buddhist perspective, sound consciousness can awaken us to a deeper, more expansive knowing. But you don't need to be Buddhist to appreciate its benefits. When we learn to open fully to sound resonance, no matter what our belief system is, we can enjoy its capacity to elicit emotion and change the habitual ways in which we meet the world. In June 2017, the Rubin Museum of Art opened The World Is Sound exhibition. New Yorkers and visitors from around the world explored how sound and hearing shape our lives and, in fact, our entire existence. The exhibition explored different dimensions of sound inspired by Buddhist philosophies of impermanence and the suffering that stems from entrenched ways of thinking. It was an invitation to "tune in" to the building and objects and occupants—all as one, all moving through space and time.

Sound Consciousness

TIME NEEDED: 7 MINUTES

LISTENING DEEPLY IS a gateway to waking up our inner aliveness. This meditation guides us to expand our field of awareness to include the changing flow of sound.

Let's take a moment now to attune to the wisdom of sound.

Let this be a return to stillness, to the mystery and magic of being.

Sit in any position that allows you to become relaxed and yet alert. It's best to close your eyes or dim them slightly.

And now begin to open awareness to any sound that meets the ear. There's no need to scan for sounds or to go seeking them. Just allow them to come to you. You might think of yourself as a satellite dish, waiting and receiving whatever comes your way. Allow the sounds to meet the stillness. Notice as they arise, exist, and then dissolve. All are impermanent, all are passing through. Sound is a beautiful way to deepen into the wisdom and insight of impermanence.

Begin to name the sounds as they appear. Naming can help you to see them as they are rather than creating a story or judging them as good or bad, right or wrong. You might name the source of the sound—"traffic" or "birds" or "fan"—or the experience of the sound—"pleasant sound" or "unpleasant sound." In time, you may notice a sense of spaciousness, no longer naming the sounds but just allowing and opening to the vibration.

Deep hearing is an experiential awakening of total consciousness, an opening to the whole of existence through mind and body. If you become distracted by the thinking mind, just return to the sounds. Let the sounds be your anchor, tethering you to the present moment.

Breathe, notice, and be.

Sound and Interconnectedness

Everything in existence vibrates, and soothing sounds have been reverberating off bells, gongs, and singing bowls for at least 67,000 years. But what can vibrational sound do for you?

In its simplest form, sound is one of the most vital ways that we communicate with each other's nervous systems. For example, the sound of your shriek, laughter, or sigh is received by the brain of your loved one and effectively dictates how their body will respond. The sounds we express change the energy we produce and reverberate throughout everything in our path. When we expose ourselves to sounds that elicit relaxation and inner calm, the ripple effect can be magical. The sounds we hear and express are an unending vibrational system, a powerful reminder of our interconnectedness.

Have you noticed how some words feel more emotionally intense and heavy, whereas others feel soothing or uplifting? We all have a list of words we don't like: "crusty," "moist," "curd," "slurp," and the all-dreaded "ointment" (ugh—the worst!) are often among them. We also have words that lift us up and motivate us beyond all reason (marketers love to use these words), including "inspired," "resilient," "authentic," and of course "glowing." Although we react to a word's meaning or association, its sound is important too. Many sound combinations seem to tap directly into a primordial element of our consciousness. For example, poetry and mantras can invoke emotional states that transcend the words themselves, enlivening a sense of connection and wonder. To hear, read, or recite a moving poem is an indescribable intimacy. And to really bring home the impact of tone and intonation, think of the last time you read a text and were convinced that the person sending the message was angry, irritated, or just plain rude only to find out later that your interpretation wasn't their intention at all. When it comes to sound, our interpretations, experiences, and genetic wiring can all come into play, leaving us feeling harmonized or unsettled.

As you move through your day, begin to collect the words that inspire or move you or elicit the kinds of emotions you'd like to wire into your neurobiology. Once you find the right words, try them on to see how they fit. Write them down and repeat them intentionally and often. Feel the vibration of the words moving throughout your body and notice where you begin to open or close. Which words would you like to come back to again and again to strengthen, soothe, or increase feelings of vibrancy? When you find the right ones, they'll become like a well-worn pair of boots walking you through the bramblebush of life.

Sound Healing

It's amazing to see what happens when we tap into the ancient healing potential of sound. Scientific studies are starting to discover the ways that music, positive words, and mantras can help relax the body and bring forward a sense of inner peace.[1] Yoga studios, hospitals, corporations, and schools are increasingly offering sound-wave treatments to help clients, employees, and students slow the heart rate, balance brain-wave activity, and calm the nervous system.

Let's look at sound baths. If you've ever finished a yoga class or a meditation with the low and slow sound frequencies of a Tibetan singing bowl or gong, you'll know the deep visceral state of relaxation they induce. But sound baths are not just a fad used at yoga retreats; they've been used for thousands of years in prayer and meditation. And only more recently has their therapeutic use been scientifically studied to better understand the impact sound has and how it helps to heal our mind-body system.

Here's the science. The sonic and wave properties of sound-healing technologies have the potential to alter our brain state to relaxing beta (normal consciousness) and theta (relaxed consciousness) wave activity. Some researchers suggest these technologies may train the brain to produce more delta waves, which have been associated with a greater sense of calm.[2] What's more, stimulating the alpha and theta waves helps us stay alert during the day and sleep more deeply at night.

So how do sounds affect overall feelings of well-being? In 2017, a group of researchers from the University of California decided to explore just that question.[3] They wanted to understand the effects of listening to singing bowls, gongs, tingshas (tiny cymbals), bells, and other Tibetan instruments. They discovered that after only sixty minutes of sound treatment, participants reported feeling less tension, anger, fatigue, and depressed mood. The sound vibration was seen to act like a butterfly net, collecting the inner chatter and leaving participants feeling deeply relaxed. While it's hard to know which part of the positive effects was the sound from the instruments and which part was the quiet solitude of lying down and meditating on a mat, the low-cost intervention left the vast majority of participants feeling a greater sense of well-being.

INTEGRATING SOUND HEALING INTO PRACTICE: MANTRA

I hadn't fully appreciated the transformative and healing resonance of sound until I had the privilege of being taught by the cherished American spiritual leader Ram Dass at the Open Your Heart in Paradise retreat in 2019. Ram Dass dedicated his life to teaching loving awareness, social consciousness, and compassionate care for the dying. He was a prophet for our times. To be with him was to experience an ocean of love so pure it opened my heart wider than I ever thought possible.

Ram Dass had had a hemorrhagic stroke two decades before, and by the time I met him his health was in significant decline. In fact, his doctors had advised those closest to him to share their final words with him just days before the retreat. However, Ram Dass seemed to will his body to allow him to stay just a little longer for us, sharing his teachings one last precious time. On the final day of the five-day gathering, Ram Dass radiated a profound presence. He gently blessed a basket of *malas* (prayer beads), each of which had a red thread from the blanket of his guru. As we received the offering, Ram Dass gazed into our eyes with genuinely life-changing love and tenderness. We sang a mantra together, and he waved his hand for us to come closer. We gathered around his frail body, and his pure, all-embracing love permeated our spirits. His loving essence, the sound of our voices carrying the spirit of the mantra, and the current of tenderness all thrived within our oneness. As the mantra peaked, something breathtaking began to take over— the current of love began to shift, moving from our hearts to his.

Mantra practice is the repetition of a sound, phrase, or set of sacred syllables during meditation or at various moments of the day. The word "mantra" is a two-part Sanskrit word: *man*, which is "mind," and *tra*, which is "transcend." It is a way to reconnect with our very essence. The words we choose are deeply personal and can go straight to our heart. These words can be chanted, whispered, or spoken internally. When we repeat anything, it strengthens the emotional patterns it elicits. Too often we repeat phrases such as "I need to be better," "I'll never be happy at this job," "My marriage is a mess." When we practice these words often enough, they become our lived reality. Thoughts inform emotions. Emotions inform reactions. Reactions inform actions, and so on, and so on, and so on.

Mantra work is a powerful way to change the neurological architecture of the mind. Mantras starve out negative pathways and create new ones. Like seeds, when mantras are watered often enough, they help us grow thought forms that bring positivity and vibrancy to our life. And the thought forms we practice affect not only how we feel but also what we authorize in our lives. The thinking mind changes our attitudinal tone, emotions, and behavior in ways we are not always conscious of, and these have an impact on our ultimate well-being. A committed practice of mantra work will transform the trajectory of your life because whatever you believe and whatever you feel in your life creates your experience.

Mantras give us wings to fly in the groundlessness. They are balms for the agitated mind and windows to self-knowing. Mantras can be repeated silently during meditation to both energize an intention and provide a focal point to cut through mental chatter. Or they can be repeated out loud to activate the calming effect of sound vibration. Chanting mantra is medicine for mind, body, and soul. The long exhales used in chanting are like a direct line to the calming parasympathetic nervous system. The brain receives the breath's message and passes the memo along to the rest of the body, letting it know there is no perceivable danger.

Mantras bring us back to the rhythm of the body—a place that is spacious in the same way that nature is spacious. And when a mantra resonates with the soul it becomes the vehicle for entering into pure awareness: the timeless moment. Whether you meditate or not, reciting a meaningful and supportive mantra can help you to relax into the moment and open to the challenges of the day with wisdom and steadiness.

MANTRA PRACTICE

To start a mantra practice, choose a meaningful word, phrase, or sound you'd like to invoke during meditation. Just think, a single well-chosen word can wake you up and call you into the moment, reconnecting you with your true self! You may need to try a few mantras until you find the one that resonates with you. Pay attention when you have a negative reaction toward a mantra. Sometimes the ego will reject what we need to open to the most.

When you've found the mantra that will best support you, you will know it immediately and feel it viscerally. Imagine that mantra as a seed that you'll nurture and nourish with attention and kindness. A forced mantra only repeats the patterns of harshness; instead,

The practices you're discovering support your vision for a life that's balanced, healthy, and free from limiting patterns. But it's going to take time. It takes perseverance and stamina to starve old patterns and ignite and breathe life into new ones. There's a word I come back to again and again when I feel myself veering off track: *Adhiṭṭhāna*. This Sanskrit word means "determined practice" and it can spark a fresh wave of determination just when you need it the most. When you feel lost or discouraged, imagine yourself as strong and steady as a mountain or oak tree, impervious to the wind and the rain, and with your strongest voice repeat the word "Adhiṭṭhāna" as you root yourself in determined practice. And keep in mind there is vast scientific evidence and 2,500 years of tradition supporting you. Keep going. I am wholeheartedly with you!

release any expectations of outcome and allow the mantra to expand your awareness, observing its resonance and opening to whatever the mantra wants to show you.

Take some time to think about the natural openings in your day. It may be easiest to add mantra work at the end of your morning meditation or at various transitions during your day. Mantra work is like muscle memory: the more often you practice, the stronger the mental pathways become. As you practice repeating the mantra, focus on expanding the diaphragm, exploring the vibration moving through and emptying the buildup of stress. The words are powerful and all-encompassing. Imagine riding the healing mantra into your heart. This is what Ram Dass taught so beautifully.

Let's practice. Begin by reading over each mantra below and notice which one resonates with you in your heart. Place the hand at the heart as you read each one and feel into the truth of your soul's needs. If one mantra doesn't speak to you immediately, make a short list of some that might fit. Take a minute or two to recite each mantra on the short list inwardly and notice which one best supports your ability to settle into awareness.

MORNING MANTRAS

My mind is awakened and I see love in everything before me

Behind the darkness is unending light

I am grateful for this body, this breath, and this life

With small steps come radical shifts

All I truly need is right here in this moment

COMPASSION MANTRAS

I am love, I am love, I am love

Peace lives in every moment

My heart speaks before my words

There is no comparison in compassion

Nothing my body is showing me can be wrong

WISDOM MANTRAS

My life is a sacred ritual

My true self already knows the answer

Self-care is not selfish—it is my birthright

Conflict is shared vulnerability

My heart space is my true home

AWAKENING MANTRAS

Every moment is my invitation to awaken

That I am separate is the illusion

There is no better place to be than right here, right now

I am free, I have always been free, I will always be free

Pain is the past, healing is the present

HEALING MANTRAS

Healing lies in every moment, and every moment is my practice

I choose community over competition

Where joy is present, anxiety cannot exist

Anxiety cannot thrive in the spaciousness of present time

Everything I see is of light, is of grace, is of oneness

EXPANSION MANTRAS

There is no time or place where light is not present

Light is the essence of who I am in truth

Peace lies in the acceptance that life is ever changing

In every moment I resee and begin again

My life is a perfect reflection of what I am here to discover

CLEARING MANTRAS

I am more than my fear, I am more than my suffering

Love dissolves fear

Compassion dissolves judgment

Grace and beauty find their way through the cracks of heartache

Letting go is as easy as exhaling

Invitation to Practice: Closed-Eye Mantra Meditation

Now that you've chosen a mantra, take a moment to settle into the body and trace your way to that quiet place within. Wherever you find yourself, take a low and slow inhale through the nose. Exhale and arrive fully into this moment.

Begin to lovingly invite the mantra into your awareness, repeating the mantra inwardly. Listen to the sound of the inner voice as the mantra arrives, exists, and dissolves, only to repeat again.

Notice the sensations and emotions that arise as you continue to recite the mantra. Relax into the words. Relax into the moment. And let the mantra open you to what's there.

If the mind becomes restless, simply acknowledge that this is a habit of the mind.

Sometimes the ego resists the change and argues. Just allow the interfering thought to be there and label it "thinking" or "unpleasant thought" or "criticism," and then simply return to the mantra once again.

Draw the mantra back into your awareness again and again. Follow the mantra beyond the limitations of the thinking mind and allow it to radiate as truth and love. Imagine riding on the wisdom of the mantra as you allow it to soothe you, strengthen you, and embody you.

After your formal closed-eye mantra practice, return to the mantra again and again throughout the day. Write it down, post it in places that you're sure to see it, and let it spark the fire for your core intention.

Om Mani Padme Hum
(The Jewel in the Lotus)

TIME NEEDED: 5 MINUTES

OM MANI PADME HUM (OHM-MAH-NEE-PAHD-MAY-HUM) is a traditional Buddhist mantra that soothes the senses, breaks through the egoic mind, and lays a pathway to an unending inner wisdom. The Dalai Lama has said that in these four words are all of the teachings of the Buddha in one.

As you chant the mantra, invite the meaning of the words into your heart.

Om: Open a gateway to inner peace and expansive awareness.

Mani: Activate inner tolerance, patience, and unconditional compassion.

Padme: Notice an inner intelligence directing you on your wise and steady path.

Hum: Rest in the spirit of your highest wisdom: enlightenment.

The choral music of this chant will tone the body, mind, and speech. As you feel the current of the mantra moving through, imagine all voices coming together in oneness and bring the mantra into the heart.

Om mani padme hum. Om mani padme hum. Om mani padme hum. Om mani padme hum. Om mani padme hum. Om mani padme hum. Om mani padme hum.

Salima's Story: Afterword

Through sound mindfulness, Salima moved more deeply into the places of pain and fear. She began to see that her reaction to sound was a messenger sending important cues when she felt unsafe or when her nervous system was flooded. Instead of blaming or judging the source of the sound, she learned to open to the sensation and even welcome it. And while the problem didn't dissolve completely, by mindfully listening and practicing compassionate acceptance she found that the gross sensations became less intense. She no longer ran from the body sensations but instead learned to hear deeply. Most importantly, she was less often in fight-or-flight mode and therefore more able to find rest, self-care, and support. Through the power of inner listening, Salima amassed the strength to enlist the help of the school's advocacy groups to address ongoing discrimination. When last we spoke, she had mobilized change across the entire university.

Top 3 Takeaways

1. The special yogic wisdom of chanting is available to everyone, Buddhist or not. Mantras send healing sound vibrations throughout the mind-body system to relax and energize all at once.

2. Sound has the ability to rebalance the body's energy frequency, releasing emotions, unblocking pathways, and improving mind-body health in ways that we are only beginning to understand. It is inexpensive and accessible to all.

3. Mantra meditation shapes the brain pathways to enliven our aspirations. Whether it is part of a meditation practice or not, reciting the day's mantra helps ground us through the challenges of the day ahead and brings us back home to our radiant self.

Journal Prompts

- What sounds do you find uncomfortable or disturbing to your sense of peace? What makes them so?

- Where do you feel the current of pleasant sounds in the body? How about unpleasant?

- What are those pleasant and unpleasant sounds teaching you about the nature of life and your reactions to it?

- Spend some time in closed-eye practice and notice the response in your mind and body as sound permeates through you. Write about the sensations, thoughts, and emotions that arise. What is the sound teaching you?

- What might change if you were to enter into whole-body listening with those in your life?

Sleep

Prioritizing Our Relationship with Sleep

*"When you have insomnia, you're never really asleep,
and you're never really awake. With insomnia, nothing's real.
Everything is far away. Everything is a copy of a copy of a copy."*

CHUCK PALAHNIUK, *Fight Club*

Shu's Story

"Sleep deprivation is a special kind of torture," she said. "I would do just about anything to sleep through a whole night." Shu had been seeing me for counseling on a weekly basis for several months, and each session began in much the same way. She would arrive just after the start of the hour, apologize profusely for being late, and enter a stream of consciousness about the overwhelming sense of hopelessness that pervaded her mind. She and her husband had recently moved from New York with their children so she could take a job at a local fashion house. They were just settling into their new home when her husband was hit on a local ski mountain by an out-of-control snowboarder. Soon after the accident he developed a seizure disorder, and while it was largely controlled with the help of anti-seizure medication, the side effects and impact of his head injury left her feeling both terrified for his safety and exhausted by the workload at home. Without any additional help, Shu was juggling work, financial pressure, driving their four kids to extracurricular activities, and attending her husband's medical appointments. It was miraculous that she was able to make it to her therapy sessions at all.

She held off tears but reached for a tissue just in case they pushed through. "I feel like I'm going to break. I'm letting things slip at work, I'm barely managing with the kids, and I don't see an end in sight," she said. "And if I get sick there's no one else to hold it together."

I could feel myself getting drawn into the hopelessness, the pressure in my own chest and sudden cloudiness in my mind telling me more about her lived experience than her words themselves. I could feel deep in my bones just how exhausted she was. "What happens in your body when you think about those words 'I feel like I'm going to break'?" I asked.

"I feel a heaviness in my body, especially my chest. And I just feel out of it, like I haven't slept in days," she replied.

"OK, let's make room for that feeling. It may help to place a hand on your chest to make contact with the heaviness you feel there. And if you'd like, you can take a low and slow breath, breathing through the nose and directing the breath to those areas of discomfort." I felt myself relaxing a little as Shu started to breathe more deeply. The tension in her body softened too. "What are you noticing now?" I asked.

"It's lifting," she said. "It's not as intense. Not as close or as fragile."

Peter Levine, a renowned trauma specialist, once said, "Anytime anyone makes a shift [addressing trauma in the body], the shift affects everyone else—on a cellular level."[1] It explains beautifully why we can feel so deeply the emotional pain of others and why we mirror each other's nervous systems.

The Magic of Sleep

Sleep is perhaps one of the most misunderstood and mysterious aspects of the human experience. The average person spends twenty-five to thirty years of their life asleep,[2] and yet most of us don't give it the recognition it deserves. We live in a culture that values busyness over rest, creating an imbalance between our sleeping and waking lives. Our lifestyles are more hurried than ever before, and high-productivity activity is not only dominating our days but now also claiming our evenings and crowding out the natural and sacred medicine of rest. And while a whole lot needs to change on a cultural level for us to resolve this societal sleep crisis, there's much that we can do personally to reclaim our sleep life.

Sleep health is also important for a rich spiritual life. Buddhism teaches that we are actually the most spiritually awake when we are asleep. The word *Buddha* comes from the Sankrit word *budh*, which means "to awaken," as in awakening from one's unawareness. Sleep is also an inherently collective experience that ties humankind together in a universal bond, but first let's look at it from a physiological point of view.

Studies have shown that people who get less sleep than they need don't just suffer the following day. If they regularly don't get enough sleep, they are at increased risk of high blood pressure, stroke, obesity, and diabetes.[3] The effects on mental health are important too: anxiety affects sleep, and lack of sleep promotes anxiety, a vicious cycle if ever there was one.[4] In addition to all of the above, the connection between sleep and overall brain health is undeniable. Sleep has an impact on our nervous system, either supporting or hindering anxiety levels, as well as on our ability to manage emotions, solve daily challenges, have clarity of mind, and show up with a freshness of spirit we all desire. While we sleep the brain goes in and out of different stages, at times bursting with brain activity. It's like overnight therapy, helping the brain to consolidate information we've learned throughout the day and processing difficult emotional experiences. It's also a time when the brain goes through a sort of deep cleaning: a watery liquid called cerebrospinal fluid (it's like a cleanup crew for the mind) flushes out proteins that can negatively affect memory and overall cognitive health.

Hormonal changes (especially decreased estrogen), technology use, light pollution, use of stimulants, and a culture of incessant stress all affect our ability to regulate the body's natural rhythms, which makes it hard to both fall asleep and remain asleep. Lack of sleep can throw our insulin levels and metabolism out of balance, compromise our immune functions, and even put us at increased risk for car accidents. Cramming for an exam or work project (maybe you're frantically trying to prepare a presentation, for example) and going nineteen hours without sleep makes us so cognitively impaired it's the equivalent of being legally drunk.[5]

Remember when you were a child how you'd fall asleep when your head hit the pillow after a day spent outside in the fresh air? Remember how good you'd feel when you woke up the next day? Imagine recapturing that experience by bringing back the joy to your sleep life. Imagine restoring and rejuvenating your mind, body, and soul with the sweetness of deep rest. It's completely within your power to do so.

Know Your Chronotype

Sleep may be a tie that binds us but that doesn't mean we all have the same sleep patterns. For example, have you ever felt annoyed by a partner or family member who just couldn't seem to get up in the morning? Or perhaps they criticized you for being a night owl? It turns out there are genetic reasons for the differences in sleep patterns. And when we think about these differences in evolutionary terms, it makes perfect sense. Our ancestors would never have survived if they'd all settled down to sleep at the same time. Who would have fought off nighttime predators? Luckily, nature was way ahead of us. She's designed each of us with our own internal body clock, known as a chronotype, which affects our sleep patterns throughout our lives. Our chronotype affects how and when our body releases the hormone melatonin, as well as our body temperature and other physiological patterns that influence the sleep-wake cycle.

Roughly 40 percent of us are naturally morning larks (people who wake early) and another 30 percent are inherently night owls (people who go to bed late); the rest of us fall somewhere in between.[6] Unfortunately, the nine-to-five schedule of corporate life or the pitter-patter of early-rising children doesn't always fit with our chronotype and its associated optimal sleep schedule. And when we're forced into a schedule that isn't a match for our body's needs, the quality of our work suffers, and the chronic sleep deprivation that comes with not honoring our body's schedule can seriously compromise our health. The mismatch that night owls face between when their body wants to sleep and the sleep schedule they're often forced to keep is so notable there's actually a term for it: social jet lag. As you learn more about your body's inherent needs, you can slowly shape your routines and lifestyle in ways that amplify your life.

The nature of our sleep style has a lot to do with circadian rhythms, the sleep-wake patterns baked into our genetics. These twenty-four-hour cycles are influenced partly by our chronotype and partly by light-sensitive cells in our retinas. These light-sensitive cells track outside information (like the amount of light coming through the window or under the door) and send a message to the brain to begin producing melatonin, the sleep-inducing hormone. The good news is that we can exert some control over this process.

Sanskrit writings have promoted light therapy for hundreds of years, and we intuitively know that our minds and bodies thrive when daylight hours are longer. Sun exposure is a natural treatment for anxiety: not only does it provide warmth to address excess *vata* (the energy associated with movement in Ayurvedic medicine), it also resets our biorhythms. Adequate amounts of light at the right times throughout the day can make all the difference to our mood, alertness, sleep patterns, and overall sense of well-being. As we age, our bodies make less and less melatonin naturally, but we can stimulate its production with exposure to natural light, especially early in the morning. That's why it's important to open the blinds as soon as you wake up. Some researchers even suggest not wearing sunglasses early in the morning.

Bedtime Rituals and Sleep Hygiene

You turn off your phone, slip into your pajamas, lower the lights, enjoy the last sip of herbal tea, and crawl into bed. The waking world is no longer your concern. You're ready to surrender to the deeply personal, if not spiritual, gateway delivered by sleep. But your mind resists, and the peace and healing that come only with deep rest seem farther away with each toss and turn of your agitated mind and body.

In my therapy practice, sleep problems are one of the most common issues my female clients bring up. Blurred lines between work life and home life, looking after children or aging parents (and sometimes both), hormonal fluctuations, high cortisol levels, tech overload, relationship stress, imbalanced diet, the pressure to be all things to all people, and a myriad of other burdens crowd out the rest so many women badly need. As the to-do list gets longer, sleep times get shorter and well-being (not to mention happiness) suffers. And yet, we must rest if we are to rise into our most vibrant and enlivened selves, fully available to what matters most to us in our lives.

It's time to reclaim bedtime and strengthen our bodies and minds through sleep.

Here are ten simple, proven techniques to connect, tap into, and cultivate deep rest:

1. Keep yourself in the dark. Blackout blinds send a clear message to the brain that it's time for sleep. Even something as seemingly innocuous as the light from a cell phone message is enough to rouse you from sleep, so scour the room and unplug any light sources before you snuggle in. And if you get into the habit of soaking up as much natural vitamin D as possible in the morning and turning down the

lights soon after dinner, your brain will serve up the right dose of melatonin to support your slumber.

2. Cutting down on caffeine is one of the easiest ways to support your body's natural rhythm and make the most of your sleeping hours. (Chapter 8 has more on the effects of caffeine.) In small doses (a quarter of a cup of coffee, for example), the effects of caffeine can be quite mild, but you can best support your nervous system by avoiding caffeine after 1:30 p.m. Check food labels when choosing your afternoon and evening foods to ensure you're not inadvertently caffeinating late in the day. And instead of coffee or hot chocolate, try having a cup of chamomile tea an hour or so before bed to relax the nervous system. Chamomile tea contains apigenin, a flavonoid found in many fruits and vegetables. It's been used in traditional medicine for centuries as an anti-inflammatory, antiviral, and antibacterial, and for its naturally calming effects.

3. Tamp down on alcohol to help you sleep better. This tip probably sounds counterintuitive if you enjoy a beer or a lovely glass of red wine to "unwind" at the end of the day, but alcohol can interfere with your breathing, cause you to wake up several times in the night (although you might not remember), and deprive you of ultra-important rapid eye movement (REM) sleep. Instead of alcohol, consider a nighttime golden turmeric latte (1.5 cups of oat milk, 1 teaspoon of grated ginger, 1 teaspoon of grated turmeric, 1 diced Medjool date, and a hint of cinnamon) and you're (ahem) golden.

4. Give yourself a few hours to wind down after doing a heavy cardio workout, so skip the late-night high-intensity interval training class. Your brain and body need a chance to recover from the surge in heart rate and endorphins (both of which make you more alert) that comes with intense exercise.

5. Put technology (smartphones, tablets, video games, TV, for example) to bed at least one hour before you hit the pillow yourself. Not only does the blue light of the screen lower your body's production of melatonin but also every ping you hear keeps your brain alert.

A single text message can increase dopamine levels (the feel-good neurochemical we all love), leaving you wanting more.

6. Try keeping a worry journal where you can note the things that are troubling you and release them from your inner monologue. The simple act of externalizing the worrying thoughts by writing them down can be cathartic and it can help you to see patterns emerging so you can address them before they become entrenched. I recommend you write in your journal at least an hour before bed to avoid ruminating as you're trying to fall asleep. Spend only 5 minutes or so jotting down three or fewer worries—it need not be an exhaustive list. As you write, ask yourself not just what is worrisome, but also why it is worrying you. Put the journal away knowing the worries have been put to rest for the night.

7. Honor the end of day with deep intention and ritual. Read a mantra or poem to yourself out loud, light a special candle, practice some yoga postures to consciously release tension from your body. Whatever you choose to do, let the ritual be unique to bedtime as a way to let the mind and body know you're closing off the day and entering into the liminal time between wakefulness and sleep. Give attention to all the small, subtle things, like drinking a cup of chamomile tea, washing your face, and mindfully turning down the lights. Do these in ways that honor and align with the needs of your mind, body, and soul.

8. Keep the temperature of your bedroom cool (between 60 and 67 degrees Fahrenheit/15 and 19 degrees Celsius).[7] The cool temperature triggers the hypothalamus in the brain to release melatonin. It can also be helpful to decompress with a warm salt bath right before slipping into bed. When the body begins to cool, it reaches the optimal temperature to induce sleep.

9. Use a weighted blanket to help soothe your body's limbic system. While the science on this subject needs more attention, one early study found that using a weighted blanket was associated with an increase in sleep time and participants found it easier to settle down

to sleep, described an improved sleep, and felt more refreshed in the morning.[8] The heavy weight of the blanket seems to mimic the benefits of deep touch therapy (or a hug), signaling a release of oxytocin (the bonding hormone) and easing anxiety.

10. Use lavender essential oil to transport you into rest. The scent has a faint powdery quality that makes it deeply soothing. It acts on the central nervous system with specific changes in the neuroreceptors associated with pain relief and relaxation.[9] According to research studies, the benefit of using lavender is in part connected to an increase in the amount of slow-wave sleep (that's deep sleep) throughout the night.[10] Whether you use a diffuser or oil roller or whether you spray lavender on your pillow, look for oil that is steam-distilled, 100 percent pure, and, ideally, organic.

While it may not be realistic to follow all of these steps—you don't want to turn optimizing sleep into another chore—begin with just one or two that might be most helpful. Adapt them to suit your circumstances. If time is an issue, for example, dim the lights, play calming music, and opt for a warm shower instead of a bath.

Once you have created an environment conducive to deep rest, what next? This is when the practice of nervous system regulation and self-honoring come together. When you slip into bed and bring the body into stillness, the mind shows you what is there. Many of us find ourselves being bombarded by thoughts, irrational fears, and unmetabolized worries from the day, which activates the limbic system and disrupts both sleep and peace of mind. To release the buildup of emotions and thoughts, try making this time before bed a ritual of sacred pause.

Start by releasing the day. I place my hands at the heart and recite this mantra in a whisper: "I give thanks to this day and all its teachings. I release that which does not serve my highest good. I welcome the solitude and deep rest for my body, mind, and spirit."

Then comes self-soothing. The breathing exercises, progressive muscle relaxation, and meditations in this book all activate calming responses that can help carry you into sleep. Turning to your practice of equanimity can do wonders to quell nighttime mental activity. It allows you to compassionately witness and accept the thoughts, emotions, and sensations without holding on to them. Equanimity gives you choice, power, and a tool to take care of your peace.

Although falling asleep may become easier with consistent use of these peace practices, you may still find yourself waking in the night. According to the Sleep Foundation, women often report more sleep disturbances than men: over two-thirds struggle to fall asleep at least a few nights per week, and almost half describe waking up feeling tired and unrefreshed.[11] If you are waking in the night, try to remain in bed and use this time as an invitation to move right back into the practice you used to guide you into deep rest. If after twenty minutes or so you are still fighting sleep, do something else—wrestling with your mind can worsen the problem. Try doing a sitting meditation, writing in your journal, or reading a book until you feel sleepy again. Just remember to keep the lights low to avoid interfering with your melatonin levels. And here's another little trick: avoid cold water if you need to hydrate. It's activating and can lead to a surge of adrenaline. And love yourself back into sleep rather than admonishing yourself or worrying about how many hours of sleep you're getting. Like anything worthwhile, sleep takes practice.

In addition to being able to sleep deeply, we also need to rest fully. Most women need at least twenty more minutes of sleep than men. Professor Jim Horne, one of the UK's leading sleep experts, points out in his book *Sleepfaring: A Journey through the Science of Sleep* that women's tendency to multitask places more demands on our brains. The more demands we make on the brain, the more restorative time it needs to function optimally. While conventional wisdom says adults need seven to nine hours of sleep, the exact amount each of us needs to become fully restored cannot be prescribed. Don't feel you need to set yourself a target. Instead, when you come to know yourself well, you'll develop a deep sense of what your mind-body system requires. And remember that duration doesn't account for sleep quality or the level of physical or emotional stress you may have experienced throughout the day. If you've been receiving texts

A LITTLE NOTE OF ENCOURAGEMENT

Don't lose heart if you're struggling to gain control of your sleep. Reclaiming rest is an act of self-care that requires great patience. It takes time to retrain ourselves for a full and deep sleep. Nothing your body is showing you can be wrong. It simply needs a little support—and it's never too late to create the conditions that support the body's natural ability to find deep and healing rest.

on your phone all day (and into the night) or you're being assaulted by traffic noise at all hours or people have been pushing your boundaries, you might be feeling so emotionally taxed that seven hours is not enough. The opposite can also be true. You may find that nine hours leaves you feeling cloudy and groggy and that seven is just perfect.

The body's internal clock likes to keep a specific schedule. Going to bed late one night and early the next throws the circadian rhythm off balance. And trying to catch up on missed sleep over the weekend doesn't work as well as you might think. You can get to know your body's internal clock by keeping a sleep log for a week or two. Chart the approximate time you fall asleep, duration of sleep, quality of sleep, and degree of rest you feel when you wake up. Then assess the patterns between the sleep behaviors and the outcome. Once you've discovered your optimal sleep schedule, aim to keep a consistent routine. It may take some planning, but do your best to slip into bed at the same time each night and resist the desire to play catchup if you didn't get enough sleep the night before. Compensating will actually do more harm than good in the long term.

If accumulating a little more sleep doesn't feel as though it will add much to your life, you might imagine it this way: adding just a half hour of sleep a night accrues to ten hours a month. That's like another whole night's sleep to power up your brain health.

Nutrients: Natural Medicine for Nervous System Support and Sleep

Certain nutrients can prime the body for the quality of rest we long for. I've listed a few of the more effective ones below. Some will be familiar to you, others less so. But the good news is that all of these nutrients are readily accessible in everyday foods. Each one has its own characteristics and brings its own benefits, but they overlap and interact with each other so you may wish to get to know them all. Begin by identifying the nutrients that are most appropriate for your current needs and add one at a time, documenting how you feel. Healing nutrients can take us from brain fog to a mental clarity unlike anything else I've experienced. They balance the nervous system and empower us through better rest, feelings of calm, and increased radiant energy. But remember that it takes time to build up a wellness reserve.

GAMMA-AMINOBUTYRIC ACID (GABA)

GABA is a naturally occurring amino acid that acts as a neurotransmitter. Sometimes referred to as "the brakes of the brain,"[12] it reduces neuronal activity in the brain and central nervous system, reducing pain and stress and leading to a greater sense of calm and serenity. Most important, though, is its ability to gear down the body and call in deep sleep.

There are four ways to increase the amount of GABA in the body.

1. It's available as a supplement in capsule form, or by eating fermented foods such as kefir, tempeh, kimchi, miso, and yogurt.

2. If that doesn't sound like your ideal tasting menu, look for it in green and oolong tea (just don't drink them later in the day, to avoid caffeine).

3. Next, whole grains, fava beans, walnuts, almonds, tomatoes, citrus, broccoli, sunflower seeds, lentils, and even cocoa (look for 70% cocoa or more) can all boost natural GABA production in the body.

4. Finally, supplements such as ginseng, kava, valerian, and passion-flower may help increase the effectiveness of the GABA already in the body. Welcome to the game-changing relationship with your local natural food store!

MAGNESIUM

Whenever I'm in a sleep struggle I take a long look at my magnesium levels, as almost all of the body's functions require it and yet the Western diet is typically lacking in magnesium-rich foods. Magnesium is one of the most common minerals on earth and has wide-ranging effects on the body. It works in tandem with melatonin (see below) which regulates our sleep-wake cycles and binds to GABA receptors. It's also a muscle relaxant and has been used to treat restless legs syndrome, also called Willis-Ekbom disease, which causes uncomfortable sensations in the legs that lead to an uncontrollable urge to move them.

There are two easy ways to increase the amount of magnesium in the body.

1. I'll talk about the importance of drinking lots of water in chapter 8, but an added benefit of drinking water is that it contains magnesium. Also, adding magnesium salts to your bath lets the body easily absorb the mineral and supports another ritual of self-care.

2. Leafy green vegetables, avocados, acorn squash, nuts, and fortified cereals are powerful natural sources of magnesium, and supplements are widely available.

MELATONIN

Melatonin is a hormone produced by the tiny pineal gland in the brain. It helps to regulate our sleep cycles. As previously mentioned, the body produces less and less of its own melatonin as we age, so in time you may need to add a melatonin supplement or take some easy steps to increase its production, such as exposing your eyes to natural light early in the morning and complete darkness at night.

Melatonin works well to reset the body's circadian rhythms when they've been temporarily disrupted, but it's not considered a permanent fix for sleep issues. I've used it as a natural antidote to jet lag many a time, and it can make travel far easier on the nervous system. It's important to use it correctly, though, and only short term. As with vitamin C, the body can metabolize melatonin quickly, before it has time to have its full effect. For this reason, I recommend slow-release melatonin supplements (preferably a grade prescribed by your doctor).

Technically, exposure to darkness triggers our body to produce melatonin, but this process also needs vitamin B6. B6 is naturally abundant in soy products, sweet potatoes, bananas, navy beans, peanut butter, and walnuts. It is also readily available in capsule form.

A word of caution: Taking too much melatonin in supplement form can inhibit the body's ability to generate its own balanced levels. This situation creates a vicious cycle of supply and demand. Fortunately, some foods can boost melatonin levels without creating this imbalance. Make melatonin part of your bedtime routine by indulging in one of the following foods at night:

1. Kiwi: Eat two kiwis one hour before bedtime.

   Why: These fruits have antioxidant qualities, contain folate, and boost serotonin, all of which help to alleviate sleep problems.

2. Tart cherries/Tart cherry juice: Drink two cups per day.

   Why: Melatonin and antioxidants for the win! Tart cherries have significantly higher levels of melatonin compared with other foods.

3. Nuts: Eat a handful of walnuts, pistachios, and cashews two hours before bedtime.

   Why: Most nuts contain a good amount of melatonin (almonds and pistachios have the highest amounts), along with omega-3 fats, magnesium, and zinc.

4. Soy milk: Drink two servings per day.

   Why: Soy milk contains isoflavones (a type of polyphenol found in legumes), magnesium, and melatonin.

5. Bananas: Eat one fruit an hour before bedtime.

   Why: Bananas are rich in L-tryptophan, an amino acid that converts to 5-hydroxytryptophan (5-HTP), which converts to serotonin and melatonin.

6. Oatmeal with pumpkin and sesame seeds: Eat one serving an hour before bedtime.

   Why: The oatmeal boosts absorption of the sleep-inducing tryptophan in the seeds. Oatmeal contains magnesium (which relaxes the muscles) and vitamin B3 (which is sleep inducing), and the oats are a complex carbohydrate, which balances energy release throughout the night.

SEROTONIN

Serotonin has been discussed widely in this book in the context of its influence on mood, but it's also shown to increase the quality of sleep by reducing rapid eye movement (REM) and sustaining the body's twenty-four-hour rhythms. New research even goes as far as to say that serotonin is not just desirable but actually essential for sleep.[13] The theory is that the brain needs "sleep pressure" in order to be tired enough to fall and stay asleep, and serotonin provides this.

There are two easy ways to boost serotonin production.

1. The amino acid tryptophan, which we get from eating protein such as turkey (known for its soporific effects at Thanksgiving!), is a key to serotonin production. For vegans, foods like seaweed and just about any kind of seed (chia, hemp, sesame, pumpkin, and flax) are great sources of tryptophan.

2. Vitamin D3, which we get through exposure to sunlight, can also trigger serotonin production.

Dream Yoga

Dream yoga can be thought of as the night shift for your practice. It's a nocturnal meditation technique that turns nightime into a healing laboratory for the mind. Essentially it allows us to explore and awaken to the many dimensions of reality by experimenting with our dreams. And it can help us soften the edges of difficult emotions and master challenges in our lives. It can help us work through inner conflict, rehearse upcoming situations we imagine will be stressful, and ultimately guide the unconscious mind toward a healing or fulfilling outcome. The idea is that by shaping our dreams we are creating new pathways to healing and opening to the impermanent nature of not only the dreams themselves but also the situations we face in the waking world every day.[14]

Nocturnal meditations begin with lucid dreaming. In this phase, we recognize that we are dreaming and we can direct the outcomes of the dream in ways that shape our experience. Some of us have been doing this instinctively since childhood; others can learn how to do it with a little practice. Here are six intentional steps to support you as you embark on this sacred practice of self-healing.

1. Set the intention to be an active participant in your dreams before you go to bed. You might gently whisper, "May my dream life be filled with discovery and may I return feeling rested and at peace."

2. Practice using dream signs (things that are out of the ordinary) to awaken you to the fact that you are dreaming. For example, you might notice someone from childhood in the dream and that can alert you to the fact that you're dreaming.

3. Begin to use the lucid dream state to change the narrative or story of the dream in ways that are uniting, healing, or empowering.

4. Use the mind as a place of positive emotional exploration rather than repeating patterns of fear or negativity. For example, if you dream that you've had an argument with your partner and you know you've been struggling with reactive anger, change your responses in the dream to shape the outcome toward a more compassionate

way. You might then extend your responses farther, practicing a sense of calm and patient awareness with other relationships that are difficult.

5. Let your imagination run wild in this unlimited plane of consciousness by guiding it to push beyond plausible scenarios. You can do this by changing the scenery, trying something you've always wanted to do, or practicing something magical (like flying) as you dream.

6. Take some time in the morning to write about your dreams: the themes, emotional undercurrents, and stories you believe your psyche is trying to understand, change, or master.

Meditating to Fall Asleep

Although formal meditation is a powerful practice to foster open, loving awareness (it's like falling awake), we can also use it to calm the mind-body system and lay the foundation for a deep and restful sleep. Meditation has been shown to not only improve sleep quantity and quality (minimizing insomnia) but also buffer us against the impact of a poor night's sleep, making it easier to get through the day. Honoring our time of rest with meditation is a gentle and wise way to transition from a busy day of doing into the healing alchemy of sleep. We invite the rest, long for it even, but too often the mind fights the stillness. The more we crave rest and the harder we try to grasp it, the more it evades us, or as writer Poppy Z. Brite observed: "The night is the hardest time to be alive and 4 a.m. knows all my secrets."[15] Meditation can gently coax us into letting go of the unending cycle of memories, plans, judgments, and yes, secrets. With the soothing wave of each breath, we release control and surrender to the spaciousness of the unending now; in other words, we move out of our own way and let nature take over. The day dissolves into a fine mist and we meet with sleep again.

The sleep meditation below draws from Vipassana, a sensation-awareness technique taught by the Buddha two-and-a-half millennia ago. Vipassana is all about living in the body, dropping the stories about it, and seeing what meets our awareness. As we scan our attention over different areas of the body, we learn to listen to what each part is telling us. It's a profound act of reconnecting with the body in the kindest way, like rediscovering an old friend with great appreciation. The approach is non-sectarian and used in schools, prisons, hospitals, and businesses across the planet. Vipassana shows us a pathway to seeing reality clearly, observing all that arises with non-judgment and equanimity. It is in the ability to bear witness to the body, reclaiming and attending to it, that we may let go and drop into the simplicity of our being.

When we bring our awareness to the body, we begin to naturally separate from the thinking mind. Through noting sensations of warmth, coolness, lightness, density, fogginess, dryness, moisture, vibration, and other sensations dancing at, beneath, and around the body, we begin to open portals to more subtle awareness and a more expansive consciousness.

There's evidence that in each moment of meditation, connections in the brain are being recalibrated and strengthened in the areas linked to the kind of calm contentment that facilitates deep rest.[16] The heart rate lowers, the nervous system is soothed, the genes involved with the inflammatory response are dampened, and stress chemicals like cortisol and epinephrine decrease.

Vipassana
(Permission to Rest)

TIME NEEDED: 14 MINUTES

FIND A COMFORTABLE place to lie on your back, perhaps on a mat if this is a formal practice or in your bed if you're using it to enter into sleep.

Close your eyes now and enter into the stillness.

If you're using this meditation as part of your daily practice, allow your eyes to open if you find yourself drifting off.

Allow the arms to rest alongside the body, palms up if that feels comfortable, and let the feet fall to the side.

In slowing down, you can now feel that which has been there all along.

Soften into your heart center and begin to attune to your inner world with great kindness.

Breathe through the nose and let each breath lift you from the weight of the day.

This is a time to give to yourself fully.

Bring your attention to the sensation at the top of the head.

Feel the sensation at the crown and trace the awareness across the surface of the skin. Watch what sensation meets you here.

Keep moving your inner searchlight along the top of the head, scanning the sensations at the surface and under the skin.

Notice the quality of each sensation as it meets your awareness. Is it warm, cool, light, dense, foggy, numb, or vibrating along the surface? Allow no part to go unnoticed.

Now keep traveling the awareness, slowly scanning down the back of the head. Notice the sensations at the back of the head, getting to know them well.

See if you can notice with a gentle and open attentiveness.

Now bring your fullest attention to the sensations at the face, with no agenda other than full presence. The forehead, eyelids, nose, and cheeks. Notice any sensations that can be detected here. Feel whatever is here to be felt at the mouth and chin. See if you can feel sensations of warmth or coolness, tingling or dullness, or whatever is here to be experienced in this area of the body. If you notice no sensation, let that be your experience too.

Bring your attention to one arm. Notice the sensations there as you travel your awareness all the way down the arm to the very tips of the fingers. Explore the sensations in the hand and fingers, sense the feelings from the inside out.

Do the same with the other arm. Scan the sensations from the shoulder all the way down the arm. Get to know that arm with all the sensations that enter your awareness.

Now begin to scan the front body, from the neck all the way down the chest and the stomach. Again, just notice if it is warm, cool, light, dense, foggy, numb, or vibrating along the surface. You're just attending to the sensations.

And now scan the back body, from the back of the neck all the way down to the hips—scanning and noticing sensations as you go.

Bring your awareness now to the top of one leg and begin scanning. Notice the sensations as you travel your awareness all the way down to the toes. With great curiosity, notice whether each sensation is warm, cool, light, dense, foggy, numb, or perhaps tingling.

Now the other leg. Notice the quality of the sensations as you travel all the way down.

As thoughts take you away into what may come or what has been, notice compassionately and just bring the mind back to the sensations of the body. The mind practices its habits, holding on to the busy blur of narratives. In time, it too will rest.

Travel the awareness back up the body, piece by piece, part by part. Leg, other leg, back body, front body, arm, other arm, face, back of the head, top of the head. Warm, cool, light, dense, foggy, numb, vibrating.

Your radiant body is already whole no matter what it has experienced. It's the perfect culmination of all the stages, cycles, and rhythms of your life. There is great worth in this time of self-honoring.

After the moon waxes, it too must wane and so it is with rest.

Breathe, notice, and be.

Shu's Story: Afterword

Stabilizing Shu's nervous system was our first priority, and we began with her sleep. The quiet time after her husband and kids went to bed had become Shu's solace. She stayed up watching Netflix or sending emails or posting on Instagram while drinking a glass of wine and taking a bite or two of her favorite chocolate. She knew she needed sleep, but the longer the evening went on the more engrossed she became in whatever she was doing. Humans are the only mammals that deliberately delay their sleep, and Shu was caught in a vicious cycle of ignoring her body's signals of fatigue and overriding them with technology and stimulants.

We discussed small but important shifts Shu could make in her habits to support sleep. She exchanged Netflix and other technology for reading a book. She began to dim the lights in the evening to signal to her body that it was time to rest. And she traded wine and chocolate for herbal tea and baked fruit. While there was no pretending that tea and fruit were as exciting as wine and chocolate, Shu was determined to reclaim her sleep. She made other adjustments too. She started using a meditation app to learn how to cue her body to relax more easily. She learned to listen to her body and nurture it compassionately. While sleep was only one part of the puzzle when it came to helping Shu return to her sense of wholeness, once her sleep was back on track her resilience shone through. It gave her the strength and support she needed to get up every day and face life's challenges head on.

Top 3 Takeaways

1. Hormonal changes, technology use, light pollution, and a cultural system of unrelenting stress all have an impact on our ability to regulate the body's natural rhythm so we can fall and stay asleep. With small changes, we have the capacity to bring back the sacred to our sleep life.

2. We can be sleep supportive by making conscious decisions about diet and lifestyle.

3. Through dream yoga, we can enter into the vast unknown of the subconscious mind and rediscover the "medicine" of the night.

Journal Prompts

- What was your experience of bedtime as a child or teenager? What beliefs did you learn then about the value of sleep?

- What are you afraid you might lose if you begin to prioritize your sleep life?

- What steps will you take to become intentional about reclaiming your sleep?

- What would you like to actively explore through the unlimited nightly adventures of dream yoga?

Sustenance

Feeding Our Well-Being

*"The food you eat can be either the safest and most powerful
form of medicine or the slowest form of poison."*

ANN WIGMORE

Lara's Story

I first met Lara shortly after her twenty-fifth birthday. She'd been
referred by her family doctor, who suggested she begin therapy to
address feelings of low mood, anxiety, and low motivation, and
chronic headaches. I'd spoken with Lara over the phone long enough
to know that she'd been away at university for over four years and
was re-adjusting to being back under her parents' roof. Needless to
say, she was finding it difficult after so many years of independence.

When Lara arrived at the office, I was pleasantly surprised.
She'd missed her previous two appointments with me and hadn't
returned my reminder email either. I also knew she'd tried three

other therapists before me and had refused to go back to each one. I had only a short time to build a connection before I too joined that list. To begin, I thought if I could better understand why she'd fired her previous therapists I might find a window into what was blocking her from staying the course.

"The therapists I've worked with just repeat back to me what I'm telling them. I know that therapists aren't supposed to tell you what to do, but it just seems to go nowhere," she explained. I took a moment to fully hear the heart of her message. Her directness showed a strength of spirit that felt encouraging to me, and the more I simply listened the more she seemed to relax into the moment. "I know we need to go over my history," she continued, "but I'm just so tired of telling the story. I had a great childhood, no illnesses, and no history of mental illness except for my grandfather who's probably an alcoholic. I get along with my parents and my brother, and coming out was basically a nonissue to my family." I learned that Lara was well supported by her friends, family, and girlfriend of two years, and she ticked all the boxes in terms of stress resiliency. Her personal history was unmarked by trauma, and until a year ago she was thriving emotionally. I could easily see why she was frustrated by the cloud of dread that was now part of her every day.

As we traced the path of her life story, she explained that her headaches and anxiety had begun at the beginning of her third year of university. She'd been taking a full course load each year, bartending at the student union, and working tirelessly with the school's gay-straight alliance group to make the campus a safer and more inclusive place. She brightened as she described the ways she'd helped change old university policies that failed to acknowledge the rights and needs of LGBTQIA+ students. Her list of accomplishments was remarkable and her quest for unconditional freedom for all was downright inspiring. I'm constantly moved by the courage of the women I meet, and Lara was a giant in her own right. But as she was running from one advocacy meeting to the next, she was ignoring one very important thing: her body's basic needs.

To sustain her energy, Lara had fallen into a steady diet of grab-and-go prepackaged meals, processed meats, simple carbohydrates, and fast food. She was regularly drinking three specialty coffees a day, or 10 teaspoons of sugar and 150 milligrams of caffeine in each drink! Whereas the American Heart Association recommends less than 6 teaspoons of sugar a day for women, Lara was consuming over 30 teaspoons in her coffee alone.[1] And most days her caffeine intake far exceeded the recommended 400 milligrams per day for adults.

I knew that to address Lara's suffering we needed to nourish her whole being. We crafted a plan that included pausing more often to mindfully attune to the body and listen to its message. She set a gentle alarm that went off every hour, and each time the bell rang she took a long and slow breath and asked, "What's happening within my body and what does it need?" She began to nourish herself emotionally with mindfulness and physically with nutrient-dense foods, herbal teas, and hot water with ginger. Lara prepared healthy meals based on a Mediterranean diet (grilled fish, legumes, fresh fruits and vegetables, olive oil, nuts) with her parents and girlfriend. She gave the same dedicated attention to her diet as she had given to her advocacy work and studies.

Your Food Story

As we discover the emotional and spiritual fulfillment of rest, meditation, creativity, mantra, connection, and other ways to enrich our inner lives, we often become aware of what our physical body is telling us too. The opposite can also be true. Our body supports us and endures unimaginable levels of physical and emotional stress, and while its resilience is astounding, our habits of neglect have a way of catching up to us. In this chapter, I'll highlight some of the most common gaps in the average North American daily menu and we'll explore ways that specific foods can restore and rebalance our mind-body system. We'll also look at how we can use mindfulness practices to honor our relationship with food. But first, let's explore the story we've internalized about food.

You've probably inherited all kinds of stories about food: good foods, bad foods, what to eat, what not to eat. And while we'll explore a variety of foods well proven to enhance the nervous system and repair and restore the health of your mind-body system, think of this chapter as an invitation to embrace a more compassionate approach to nourishing yourself. We'll lean into the science of holistic nutrition and confront the stories that keep us perpetuating patterns of shame and feeling unworthy.

Our relationship with food can show us exactly where we are with ourselves and our culture, if we let it. The food we prepare is layered with emotional connections, family traditions, stories about ourselves, our worth, and patterns of self-nurturing or self-harm. So many of we women long for permission to love ourselves, to nourish ourselves, and to rewrite our story about sustenance and our body. If this idea sounds familiar to you, let me invite you to renew your relationship with food and the ways you care for your powerful, life-sustaining female body. And if it doesn't resonate with you? Join us as we learn more about nourishing our physical, mental, and emotional selves.

I also want to encourage you to reclaim the pleasure of eating. While nutrition is of course critical to our health, embracing ourselves fully means taking a more holistic approach to the ritual of eating, whether we eat alone or with other people. Food can be deeply intimate and life affirming when we approach it with openness. A first step toward making this positive shift is knowing what you bring to the table (so to speak) in terms of emotional patterns of eating.

Rewriting Your Food Story

TIME NEEDED: 9 MINUTES

TAKE A MOMENT now to become still and begin to listen to the inner signals of the body. Ask the body what it most needs in this moment. It may need a low, slow breath or a long sigh, or it may want you to move the hand to the heart in an expression of self-compassion. Notice where the body is holding tension and send the breath into those areas. Use the breath to relax into the body with kind, open attention.

The body may want to move or stretch or hydrate. It may feel hunger. Give it the time and patience it deserves as it speaks to you. Use this time for inner listening and attending to the messages the body is sending you. If you're not sure what the body is trying to say, allow that too. Allow yourself to be in the not-knowing.

Now bring your awareness to one of the strongest memories you have of eating or preparing food as a child or teenager. Notice which memories come forward automatically and focus your attention on just one. Settle into the scene and observe the reactions in the body as you do. Notice any changes in the breath and any places of holding or letting go.

Look now to see how old you are in that scene and rediscover how you felt at that time. How did you feel about your body at that age? Begin to scan that scene to see who else is there. You may notice friends or family members, or perhaps you're alone. Are you internalizing any messages about your body or about food from those around you? If so, what are they?

Again, scan the body and notice its reaction to this scene. Allow the sensations, emotions, and thoughts to exist in your awareness with great acceptance and compassion. You may even find yourself feeling curious about the ways this younger version of yourself began to relate to her body and food itself.

Connect now with your wisest self, that inner knowing and vast intelligence that is available to you always. You might sense it as an inner light glowing from the inner vision of the mind. Find it. Feel it. Trust it. Notice now if there are any messages that your wise self wants that younger self to know. Or you might ask your younger self what she most needs from this wise being. Notice what feels natural and authentic here. She may need to talk or get angry or cry. If she wants, let her explore the kitchen cupboards with curiosity and boldness. Let her open the fridge and intuitively sense what she most wants: touching, smelling, and tasting. Teach her the way of joy and awareness as you explore what sustenance truly means, rewriting any negative stories of body and food together.

Before you return, remind your younger self that you'll check in on her from time to time. You can also invite her into your present life by creating a seat for her at your table (real or imagined). Include her as you cook in your kitchen, and take her with you as you meander through the grocery store, or pick out vegetables at the farmers market, and explore the beauty of food together.

The Natural Healing Capacity of Food

The story of the Buddha goes that Sujata, the daughter of a village headman, saw Siddhartha's suffering as he sat under the bodhi tree. She presented him a bowl of sweet milk rice. Sujata's kind offering gave Siddhartha the nourishment and strength he needed to awaken, and so Buddhism was born. A steaming bowl of soup, beautifully roasted root vegetables, or a nut butter slathered over an apple can offer the energy to heal, focus, create, learn, cry, laugh, and awaken. To journey through our lives in an empowered way requires rich sustenance—nature's medicine in the form of nutrient-dense foods.

As we enter into the practical and functional task of making food choices, allow me to bring in the scientific dharma of nutrition. The Western way is to look for the miracle meal plan that will transform our well-being. While I would love to provide that for you, experience has shown me that starting with one or two changes at a time and building on a foundation of consistency is the recipe for long-term gains in our well-being. The more often we approach those small changes with an open inquisitiveness, the more we are moved toward choices that bring joy and vitality to every aspect of our being, including the emotional, mental, physical, and spiritual. This approach is the antithesis of following meal plans or diets, which help us achieve short-term goals such as weight loss, but are ultimately unsustainable. They leave us feeling guilty, hungry, and caught in a push-pull relationship with our body and food. Instead, we can encourage ourselves to explore nutritious foods and our bodies with an adventurous and open spirit. We'll track and listen to the subtle signs of what works and what doesn't work and teach the body to trust in our ability to care for it once again.

Loving the Gut

We know that our sense of happiness is heavily influenced by our activity levels, sleep health, and neurochemical balances and the ways we relate to the thinking mind, but what about gut health? The gut is the name for our gastrointestinal tract, a continuous feeding tube that starts with our mouth and extends all the way to the anus. Its primary functions are to absorb nutrients, communicate with the immune system, and prevent inflammation. Some theorists have begun to call the gut the "second brain" since it's the only organ in the body with its own independent nervous system and it's strongly linked to the quality of our mood and perceptive awareness.

According to the American Psychological Association, the gut is a sophisticated network of neurons exerting a potent influence over our emotional well-being. While research on the gut microbiome—the community of bacteria and other microorganisms in our gut—is still in its infancy, we do know that these bacteria produce approximately 95 percent of the body's supply of serotonin.[2] More than 100 million neurons are present in the cells that line the gut walls, especially in the small and large intestine. When we feel what we unthinkingly call our gut instincts, or butterflies in the stomach, they are well worth listening to! This communication system between the gut and the brain is bidirectional; in other words, the signals can start in the gut, the brain, or both. Our emotions and mental tone therefore affect gut health and vice versa.

The coming and going of information from the gut regulates the digestive tract. Under regular circumstances, the bacteria breaking down food particles send messages to the vagus nerve that all is well and that digestion can occur. The vagus nerve relays this information to the brain, which gives a thumbs up and sends blood to the gut so the digestion of important nutrients can take place. When we're under stress, however, the sympathetic nervous system communicates the need to prepare our bodies for danger. In the gut, it sends the message to divert energy and blood supply from processing food. The vagus nerve shuts down and anti-inflammatory molecules cannot be released. And food particles are not broken down into their component vitamins, minerals, fatty acids, and antioxidants for proper absorption. Over the long term, chronic stress can lead to nutrient deficiencies even if we've drawn from excellent food sources. Stress can also change the number and types of bacteria in the gut. And if the wall of the lining is weakened due to an inactive vagus nerve, unwelcome substances such as metabolites, toxins, and unwanted bacteria leak in and make their home in the gut. The gut truly calls the shots—messages sent from the gut up are more powerful than those from the brain down.[3]

Foods to Support Gut Health

Life is an incredible system of micro and macro environments, an intricate and interconnected web of life-sustaining forces. The earth has an incredibly rich landscape of biodiversity with everything it needs to thrive under the right conditions. The same can be said for our gut microbiome. If we nourish ourselves with foods to encourage a diverse and beneficial population of bacteria, our inner landscape is left healthy, resilient, and life supporting.

Some key superfoods nurture and nourish the gut microbiome in ways that transform it into a lush garden.[4] And even better, these foods are commonly available, so you won't need to seek out specialty grocery stores and spend the equivalent of a small mortgage to stock up.

Almonds: a prebiotic that is best eaten finely ground to support absorption

Apple cider vinegar: full of pectin, a prebiotic that flushes out pathogens and toxins

Bananas: a prebiotic that reduces inflammation

Cruciferous vegetables: nutrient-dense greens, such as kale, broccoli, cabbage, and Brussels sprouts

Fiber-rich foods: apples, carrots, almonds, rolled or steel-cut oats, brown rice, quinoa, berries, beans, pears, and other foods rich in fiber that decrease gut inflammation and promote good gut bacteria

Kefir: a fermented milk drink much like a thin yogurt that is high in nutrients and probiotics. Water kefir has similar benefits.

Kimchi: a Korean pickle that's as delicious as it is gut enhancing. Because it's fermented, it brings good bacteria to your intestinal tract.

Kombucha: a fermented tea loaded with enzymes, organic acids, and natural probiotics. Kombucha typically contains one-third the amount of caffeine as coffee. Make sure to look at the list of ingredients, though, as some brands load their product up with sugar.

Onions: a vegetable with sulfur-containing metabolites that reduce inflammation

Sauerkraut: naturally fermented cabbage that restores the balance of bacteria in the gut

Soybeans: fermented soybean products like miso and tempeh are rich with probiotics

Stimulants: Energy Thieves

Stimulants have become our Western world's go-to for regulating natural feelings of fatigue, stress, and other symptoms of internal discomfort. Instead of honoring fatigue with rest or opening ourselves to difficult emotions, we reach for a cup of coffee, glass of wine, or giant chocolate chip cookie (my personal favorite), often without thinking about what we're doing. These stimulants may give us a temporary surge in mood and energy, but that surge is often followed by anxiety, irritability, or low mood. So the stimulants we use to lift us up instead rob us of the sustained energy we need to thrive.

When you start weaning yourself off stimulants, you may get some pushback from the egoic mind, which is trying to convince you that you need that espresso shot to make it through the afternoon energy dive or that it's a much deserved "treat." If this happens, pause and ask yourself, "What am I truly feeling, where in the body am I feeling it, and what does my body really need?" In time, you may notice yourself resisting automatic patterns and using the craving as an invitation to practice mindfulness and equanimity, simply observing the emotions with openness and not wishing them away.

Coffee, that morning staple for so many of us, is a powerful drug in many ways. It has been shown to inhibit the region of the brain that regulates anxiety while it overstimulates the region that alerts us to threat. Although cutting out your coffee habit may seem unthinkable, decreasing your intake over time is one of the simplest (and safest) ways to support your nervous system.

Here are a few other stimulants you might want to avoid.

Alcohol: Although alcohol may initially act as a pick-me-up, it's actually a depressant linked to increased cortisol levels and reduced serotonin. You may feel a short-term boost in both mood and energy if you drink alcohol, but try to keep your consumption to a minimum. The maximum recommended amount for women is ten standard drinks (5 oz/142 milliliters of wine) per week, though even a small amount of alcohol can affect your awareness. If you've ever gone alcohol-free for several weeks or months at a time, you may have sensed the often dramatic improvement in mental clarity, sleep quality, and mood. So if it's the ritual of a drink that you look forward to, take out your most beautiful glass and fill it with low-sugar kombucha or sparkling water with a splash of juice instead.

Artificial sweeteners: Many studies have drawn a link between artificial sweeteners (for example, aspartame, sucralose, and saccharin) and anxiety. They are particularly implicated in destabilizing gut health.[5] For a sweet treat, snack on berries, dark chocolate, dates, or baked apples.

While it's not easy to break habits that may have been with you throughout your lifetime, and it's challenging to make nutritious food choices when time is limited, slow and steady wins the race. Remember, with each small step you're on your way to creating radical shifts in your health. Life is a master class in self-knowing and self-nurturing—and that takes time.

Caffeine: Aim for no more than 400 milligrams a day (the equivalent of four standard cups of coffee)[6] or switch out your caffeinated drink for herbal tea, chicory root, chaga, reishi, golden milk (ginger, cinnamon, turmeric, cardamom, vanilla, and a minced date), or lemon and ginger in hot water.[7] Less-obvious sources of caffeine include products with coffee or matcha flavoring (such as ice cream or yogurt), chocolate, energy bars, weight-loss supplements, and even some brands of kombucha. As a rule, check the labels of products branded "energy"—many of them are loaded with caffeine.

Sugar: The surge and then crash in blood sugar levels after you've enjoyed a sugary treat makes sugar a major contributor to symptoms of anxiety, irritability, and mood swings. Plummeting blood sugar levels after eating sugar can lead to shakiness, sweating, rapid heartbeat, and even panic attacks. Since sugar is hidden in many of the foods we eat, it's not always easy to avoid. (This is where I get worked up thinking about the number of kids choosing foods they believe to be healthy, such as yogurt, soups, and pasta, and to which manufacturers have often added large amounts of sugar.) This is as true of many products in the health-food stores (organic sugar is still sugar) as it is of products in standard grocery stores. Again, if you're buying packaged foods, reading the labels is one of the best ways to protect yourself from high sugar content. Look to avoid or cut back on white and brown sugar, corn sweetener and corn syrup, honey (yes, honey), malt sugar, molasses, and anything ending in "ose" (glucose, lactose, fructose, dextrose, and so on).

Keep in mind that sugar also shows up naturally in carbohydrates, like fruits, vegetables, and grains, but these are an excellent steady source of energy since the body digests them slowly. There's an immense difference between naturally occurring fructose (say in an apple or a banana) and the processed form. First, the amounts of fructose in fruits and vegetables are far lower than in processed foods and the fiber slows its absorption, supporting liver function. Fruits and vegetables also deliver lots of antioxidants and essential minerals. So opt for a serving of plant carbohydrates as a replacement for that sugary snack and stabilize blood sugar levels by eating protein every few hours.

Invitation to Practice: Tracking Stimulants

For the next few days, write down the stimulants you find yourself reaching for (caffeine, alcohol, sugary foods, etc.), the feelings you have at the time, the time of day, and the circumstance (at work during a meeting, at home just before bed, etc.). While the patterns to your stimulant cravings may not always seem apparent, they are likely linked to a nutritional need, an emotional need, or both. Feeling unfocused, tired, bored, anxious, or downright hungry can all lead us to succumb to cravings.

Once you've identified the times of day or circumstances that trigger your cravings, plan a replacement behavior. For example, if you're reaching for a sugary snack because you're hungry, stabilizing your blood sugar levels with a complex carbohydrate or protein every few hours will prevent cravings. And if you find yourself reaching for wine because you're feeling anxious at the end of the workday, schedule a walk outside, meditate, or do another activity that helps soothe your nervous system. If you crave sugar at the end of the day and you've linked it to feeling bored, take a moment to open to the feeling and then build in some time to spend on something you've always wanted to learn to refocus your attention. In other words, when we respond to the body's signals by feeling them more fully and accurately addressing the body's need, we can begin to rewire and balance our nervous system for greater health.

Nutrients to Support the Nervous System

What we feed our bodies can have a dramatic impact on the health of our nervous system. Foods rich in vitamins, healthy fats, anti-oxidants, and minerals protect the brain and minimize the amount of time and energy the nervous system spends in catabolic mode (processing and breaking down molecules). Let's take a look at the foods that play the biggest role in enhancing and balancing the nervous system.

DIETARY FIBER

In recent years, there has been growing interest in the ways in which dietary fiber can support gut health. Specifically, gut bacteria ferment dietary fiber to produce short-chain fatty acids which minimize symptoms caused by chronic stress.[8] Fiber also minimizes inflammation in the brain, which is found to be more pronounced in those struggling with anxiety.[9] The amygdala is one part of the brain particularly affected; when the brain has inflammation, the amygdala becomes destabilized, increasing anxiety. Stabilizing the microbiome through foods rich in dietary fiber helps protect the amygdala, and in turn, your peace of mind. Some delicious sources of fiber are black beans, brown rice, apples, blackberries, peas, barley, strawberries, raspberries, bananas, avocados, lentils, cruciferous vegetables, and bran.

MAGNESIUM

Magnesium plays a critical role in the regulation of at least 300 enzyme systems that regulate biochemical reactions in the body, and yet it can be widely lacking according to recommended standards (Health Canada recommends 250 milligrams for women per day).[10] For many of us, a typical Western diet of foods high in fats, sugar, and simple carbohydrates often replaces green leafy vegetables, nuts, and seeds that are high in magnesium and also reduces our ability to absorb this life-sustaining mineral. People with underlying health issues like gastrointestinal problems, celiac disease, or Crohn's disease, or who are insulin resistant are most at risk of magnesium deficiency. Women who drink too much alcohol are also at higher risk, given the impact of alcohol on liver function and the liver's key role in regulating our magnesium levels.

While it's relatively rare, I've known women with low levels of magnesium to struggle with leg cramps, fatigue, irregular heartbeat, numbness, nausea, or panic attacks. Once their magnesium levels were corrected, they returned to their healthiest selves. Magnesium is key to regulating stress, relaxing the muscles, and alleviating chronic tension. Unfortunately, when we're under high levels of stress we lose magnesium stores through urine and sweat. Vitamin D3 and magnesium are a health-producing team, with magnesium playing a role in either boosting D3 levels when they become depleted or bringing them down when they get too high. And if your magnesium levels are too low, your D3 may be deficient as well.

Here's the good news: Magnesium is available in many forms, as a nutritional supplement in capsule or powder form (do consult with your doctor first) and through many delicious foods. Good sources include green vegetables, dark chocolate, almonds, bananas, legumes, avocados, cashews, peanuts, buckwheat, quinoa, and edamame. And while these foods do contain magnesium, we need to eat a lot of them to get our required daily dietary intake, so supplements are well worth considering.

OMEGA-3 FATTY ACIDS

Few nutrients have been studied, and have had their value supported, as strongly as omega-3 fatty acids. Fatty acids are the building blocks of the fat in the body and the foods we eat. During digestion, the body breaks down dietary fat into fatty acids, which are absorbed into the blood. Two essential fatty acids are omega-3s and omega-6s. Omega-3s play an important role in our diet and contribute to the basic health of all the cells in the body.

One of the strongest studies to date looked at the impact of omega-3s in a randomized controlled trial of healthy young adult medical students (both male and female). Those who were given omega-3s showed significantly lower levels of both inflammation and anxiety.[11] In fact, those given omega-3s were 20 percent less anxious than their peer control group. A meta-analysis of nineteen studies found an overall reduction in anxiety among participants who were given high doses of omega-3s (up to 2,000 milligrams per day).[12] While more studies are needed, research to date suggests that omega-3s are an important component in healing the anxious brain, likely because of their anti-inflammatory properties.[13]

You'll find omega-3s in Brussels sprouts, walnuts, flaxseed, chia seeds, hempseed, algal oil, and spirulina oil.

TRYPTOPHAN

Best known for its sleep-inducing effect, tryptophan is an important amino acid for ensuring the body has enough of the feel-good neurochemical serotonin. Amino acids create proteins that help neurotransmitters send messages to and from the brain. The body cannot produce tryptophan, so it has to be ingested. The body then synthesizes tryptophan to produce serotonin, melatonin, niacin, and other mood-regulating compounds. Keep in mind that turkey isn't the only source of tryptophan. Leafy greens are rich in this all-important amino acid. Some other good sources of tryptophan are butternut squash, soybeans, walnuts, oat bran, cacao powder, cashews, and dried peas.

SELENIUM

Selenium is an often-overlooked trace mineral critically important to immune health, cognitive health, minimizing the risk of cancer, and thyroid health—it's important to both the production and regulation of thyroid hormones.[14] The body needs selenium to get the most out of antioxidants because they work in tandem to fight inflammation and damage from free radicals (naturally occurring atoms in the body that can damage cells). And selenium and iodine also work together, so take a look at your iodine levels too if you're deficient in selenium. Selenium is easy to include in your diet through Brazil nuts, mushrooms, soybeans, and sunflower seeds. If you're getting enough selenium through your natural food sources, it's best not to overdo it. In most cases a supplement is unnecessary and can pose a health risk, especially for those with autoimmune disease (it has immunostimulant effects), if you exceed daily recommended amounts.

Invitation to Practice: Mindful Eating

Mindful eating guides our whole being in selecting, preparing, and eating food. It immerses heart, mind, and body in the fullest experience of the colors, scents, textures, and flavors of foods. Mindful eating transforms self-criticism into self-nurturing and opens us to the innate wisdom of our body and nature's medicine itself.

1. Before you start eating, take a moment to pause, feel the breath as it enters and leaves the body, and begin to listen to the sensations within the body. Relaxing into the moment will support the nervous system and prepare the body for the task ahead. A calm body will more willingly process the food you're about to eat and absorb the nutrients more fully.

2. Now begin to really take in the qualities of the food before you, noticing its shape, color, texture, and smell. See if you can bring an attitude of openness and nonreaction as you get to know the foods. You might imagine that you've never seen or tasted these foods

before. Consider all that occurred for this meal to make it to your table: where and how the food was grown, how it was prepared, who contributed.

3. Slowly begin to eat, chewing mindfully with small bites and engaging all of the senses. Savor the moment and offer your fullest presence to the food and your body. Notice the quality of the relationship between you.

4. Bring curiosity and kind attention to whatever arises in your thoughts, emotions, and sensations, and openly observe the changing tastes, textures, and temperature of the food. Notice the body's response to the food.

5. Once you've finished eating, you might take a moment to reflect on the ways you'd like your food choices to support your local and wider environment.

Mindful eating can easily become your devotional practice of self-care and compassion. It's available to you each and every time you sit down for a meal.

How to Quench Anxiety

If I asked you to turn inward and imagine a place that connects you with a feeling of deep inner peace, what would you picture? A beach? A lake or stream? How about a light misty rain or a cleansing bath? If you're like most people I've worked with, your internal healing image probably included water. We were born from water. We took our first breaths with water. And we often return to water to bring peace to our mind and body. In our deepest knowing, we understand that water is sacred. It's so much more than another commodity we can control, buy or sell, order up as flat or bubbly, or allow to spill into our drains and ditches with little regard. The truth is water is one of the most powerful examples of our oneness with nature and it is healing beyond measure.

Water is a great purifier both physically and emotionally. It cleanses and primes the body for its highest well-being: it transports oxygen, provides and supports the absorption of much-needed nutrients (like sodium, calcium, and magnesium), protects our vital organs and joints, regulates body temperature, detoxifies, and moisturizes the air in our lungs. Every cell in our being requires water, and 60 percent of the human body is water. So when we fail to replenish the water we lose through breathing and sweat and urine, dehydration triggers fear in the mind-body system. The body believes it's under threat, stress chemicals like cortisol increase, and the fight-or-flight response kicks into gear. And yet, years of stress and overfocusing on the mind have clouded our intuitive ability to listen to our body's natural wisdom. We chronically ignore the body's simple need for hydration.

While our body's life-preserving alarm signals are irrefutably remarkable, they can often be delayed. For example, when we are experiencing thirst, we are already dehydrated.[15] Even mild dehydration can create an internal imbalance: a loss of as little as 1.35 percent of our fluid levels can mean a decline in mood, energy levels, and mental clarity, according to studies from the Human Performance Laboratory at the University of Connecticut.[16] To avoid headaches, constipation, irritability, sleepiness, and confusion, turn to water.

Especially important is to hydrate as soon as you wake up, as the body loses up to four cups of water while we sleep. If you don't hydrate first thing in the morning, it can be hard to catch up throughout the day. Leaving a large glass of water on your nightstand, beside your toothbrush, and on your breakfast table are simple tricks to help you remember. During the day, place carafes of water in places you're likely to notice (your bedside table, desk, etc.) so you hydrate before you feel thirsty. Another good tip is to pay attention to your urine. If it's dark or pungent, you aren't hydrating enough. Each day, aim to drink a half to an ounce of water for every pound you weigh. In hot weather and during exercise, aim for an ounce rather than a half ounce.

And as another way to bring in the sacred pause, you might take a moment to honor the gift of clean water before you hydrate. Ask it to heal you, soothe you, and support you with infinite vibrance.

Finding Inner Calm
through Water

TIME NEEDED: 7 MINUTES

THIS MEDITATION IS beneficial for releasing stress and allowing peace to flow through the body.

With each in-breath, let the healing current flow into those places of holding, tension, and gripping. With each out-breath, let it soften, soothe, and release places of tension.

Let's begin.

Hold a small bowl of warm water in front of you at the heart center and take a moment to allow the mind and body to fully connect with the water—yourself and the water as one.

Turn inward, allowing your eyes to close, but not completely.

Elongate the spine and shine the heart upward to the sky.

Inhale with a low and slow breath, suspend the breath, and exhale fully.

Again, inhale with a low and slow breath, suspend the breath, and exhale fully.

Begin to find the calm that is your natural state.

Relax into the present moment with each breath, the water supporting you. Notice the way the water moves and swirls in the bowl. You might feel the steam as it meets your skin.

And now begin to imagine yourself as an ocean wave drawing away from the sand with each inhale.

Pause as it fully retracts.

And then greet the sand again with each exhale.

Notice now the natural movement of the breath receding and flowing back in.

What is breath but a wave, arising and passing through the force of earth and moon?

Let it fill what is empty and move what is blocked.

Let the water be the peacemaker of any held pain, so soothing and calming.

Water brings balance. It is the protector of the body: cleansing, purifying, nourishing.

Where there is water there is life. May it enliven you with each breath.

With each inhale, let the waters shore up that which you most need.

And with each exhale, let the waters release what no longer serves.

Each healing wave washing through you, within you, radiating and rippling out with the rhythms of the breath and the body.

Let it soften and soothe your heart.

Let this same peace flow to anyone you've ever met, anyone you've ever known.

Let it flow to everyone on this earth and beyond.

Breathe, notice, and be.

Lara's Story: Afterword

In just a few days of her following the health guidelines for sugar intake, Lara's headaches began to subside. And while making the dietary changes wasn't always easy, Lara's commitment to healthy eating was paying off in spades. Her skin color, energy, and mood were brighter every time she returned to my office. Last I saw Lara, she had just started law school and was radiantly healthy, mentally and physically.

Top 3 Takeaways

1. Our bodies are wise beyond measure. They know what they need to thrive. When we support our body with nature's medicine, we empower it to heal and strengthen.

2. Slow, steady changes are the key to success when it comes to making sustainable dietary changes.

3. Mindful eating is a way to rediscover one of the most pleasurable aspects of life. It opens us to our inner cues and lights a path for self-nurturing.

Journal Prompts

· What do you remember about mealtimes as a child or adolescent?

· What stories have you held about food and your body? What are you truly ready to let go of?

· What signs from the body are you ignoring? In what ways are you compassionately listening?

· When do you reach for caffeine or other stimulants most often? What emotions are you usually having at the time?

· What steps are you willing to take to more fully support your body's needs?

Nature

Lessons from Mother Nature

"We need the tonic of wildness... At the same time that we are earnest to explore and learn all things, we require that all things be mysterious and unexplorable, that land and sea be indefinitely wild, unsurveyed and unfathomed by us because unfathomable. We can never have enough of nature."

HENRY DAVID THOREAU, *Walden: Or, Life in the Woods*

Artemis's Story

Artemis is my dream client. She is the Greek goddess of the wilderness, daughter of Zeus and Leto. She's fiercely independent, listening only to the whispers of the wild. She's a protector of all women, reigning with rage as she battles the harm of oppression. Artemis is the woman within us who attunes to the rhythm of nature itself. Your inner Artemis is wise. She understands that to liberate women is to also free the souls of men. She lights a fire in your belly. To allow and deepen into the Artemis within is to discover the wisdom in her fury. Where you have denied anger, she has participated in it. Where you have repressed, she has given voice. She is fierce and loud and disruptive as she bellows the sound of the collective voices of all women. She is unafraid.

She guides you as you walk through the forest decompressing from the tension and struggles of the day. She speaks to you as you sink your hands into the soil and when you harvest and forage the seasonal fruits and vegetables from your garden or flower boxes. Artemis takes her place beside you when you are lost in fear and urges you toward solace and strength in the arms of nature. She visits you in your dreams, where she leads you to the mountains, waterfalls, and meadows filled with wildflowers.

Artemis is also part of you. She is the part that knows that when you open yourself to nature, all of the striving and seeking and self-criticism fall away. She is encoded in your being, a perfect reflection of a universal essence, the mysterious and powerful forces that connect you to the deepest part of yourself and everything around you.

The Artemis Within

TIME NEEDED: 8 MINUTES

LET'S TAKE A moment now to turn inward. Sit in an upright and comfortable way. When you're ready, close your eyes and begin to listen deeply. Be aware of the breath and the body settling into this moment. Let the eyes be soft. Relax at the shoulders.

With this embodied presence, breathe in any quality that might support you, strengthen you, or nourish you emotionally. And breathe out any barriers and blocks that keep you from your highest well-being. Imagine letting go of all of the attachment to hurt and sadness and longing and pain, or any other emotions that arise.

Let the breath be the transformation.

Bring a gentle awareness to your inner world and be aware of yourself as light, illuminating from the inner vision of the mind, radiating as essence throughout the whole body. Take some time to really sense the truth that there is an unlimited self that exists beyond the body and mind.

After a time you begin to notice, far off in the distance, a beautiful column of light, a roadway extending to the rivers and forests, oceans and mountains. And as you listen, you begin to hear the wise voice of Artemis calling you back to the way of nature, the life-sustaining source that heals and nourishes.

You can see her sitting and waiting, as strong as she is sage. She sees the ways you've struggled, searching for answers where they cannot be found. She knows of your fear and fatigue and of the sadness you've tucked away in places unknown. Let her eyes meet yours and fully take in her gaze.

Now slowly that being of exquisite strength begins to move toward you. Feel her energetic presence and nature's medicine expressing itself through her. She moves even closer until her radiant light enters your heart. Just notice what it's like as the energy of her loving heart permeates yours.

Breathe deeply and now slowly let that light grow in size until it fills your entire body. Illuminating now through the head, the torso, the arms, the legs. And now in the skin of your body is this radiant being. A being of natural grace who sees clearly her strength and resilience.

Living as one organism, a being of fierce compassion and wisdom. An aurora of beautiful light, illuminating the way for healing on this planet. Shining out at all of the people and creatures who are at the edge of fear or longing or have lost their way. Allowing your heart to touch theirs. Blanketing them in healing light, because at this moment you can know yourself to be of strength and wisdom, and of nature's radiance.

Breathe, notice, and be.

Bringing Nature In

Mother Nature. She is innately compassionate, supportive, and intuitive. She knows what we most need and gives it openly, selflessly. Nature also teaches us to slow down, to observe, and to feel deeply. Turning toward nature isn't about escaping or separating from the truth of the moment. Instead, it teaches us to get out of the mind and into the body. A return to nature is a return to the fullest expression of the true self.

I live near a park called Pacific Spirit that has dozens of beautiful walking trails through the rain forest, where my dog, Lloyd, can

A LITTLE NOTE OF ENCOURAGEMENT

The egoic mind is very skilled at pointing out where we've faltered or are falling short (as if that's even a thing). Counteracting this mind habit takes two things: mindfulness and compassion. Transforming our lives isn't a straight line. We seed, we grow, we bloom, and the old self dies, over and over again. So count the signs of growth (literally tally the positive actions by writing them down throughout the day) and teach the mind to pay attention to them. At the same time, honor those times of difficulty knowing they're a necessary stage of growth. This balanced view can offset self-criticism and build confidence in acknowledging the many small but cumulative steps you're taking throughout the day to build a lifetime of well-being. Look for the signs you're healing, growing, and expanding, and love equally those times of retraction.

explore and I can feel the restorative beauty and ancient wisdom of the cedar trees. I recognize how fortunate I am. Not all of us have a spirit-affirming rain forest in our backyard—which is why it's so important that we protect our forests and fortify our cities with green space. Getting back to nature can be as simple as opening the car window while driving down a leafy street or finding a patch of grass to have lunch on—the important thing is to make it a regular part of self-care. Examples of nature's beauty are everywhere: in a snowflake, in a flower, and in the seasons themselves. And while each of us may at times doubt and question our worth, nature is a reminder that we are all part of a sacred awareness.

I, too, have become lost in my mind for long periods of time, awakening again and again from my own stupor. I'm baffled each time by the ways in which the mind takes me away into planning and organizing, and narratives that have nothing to do with the truth of the moment. At times the mind patterns can be unbearable.

When the quietness of nature brings me back into awareness once again, I can't help but feel grateful. Writer Margaret Bates once said, "Between a human and a tree is the breath. We are each other's air."[1] I feel an unlimited kindness in the trees.

Suzanne Simard is a professor of forest ecology who has conducted a great deal of research on the very same forest that I walk in each day, and she describes an intuitive wisdom to trees that truly boggles the mind. According to her research, as trees live side by side for hundreds of years they learn and adapt their behaviors, perceive and recognize one another's needs, give warnings, and even remember the past.[2] She describes that trees have traits that are ascribed to the essence of civil societies: trees have an intelligence that is innately social, healing, and cooperative.

Invitation to Practice: Walking Meditation

Walking meditation is meditation in action where the moving body becomes the anchor of awareness. Once today, and every day after, extend your meditation practice to walking mindfully in nature, whether that means a hike in the forest or just watching the pigeons as you walk through town. Walk slowly, intentionally, focusing 25 percent of your attention on the breath and the rest on the sensation of movement in the body and the senses. Breathe through the nose. Relax your left hand over the right one and lower the gaze, resting it six feet in front of you. Walk slowly and attune to the sights, smells, and sounds of nature. In time you can vary your speed, going from mindful walking to mindful running. But remember, you're not trying to get anywhere. So feel the hum of natural life moving through and open with gratitude to the simple beauty around and within you.

Nature by Design

Even in the world of architecture and design, the natural world is having a moment. Biophilic design (the building industry's approach to bringing people and nature together) is everywhere, from green roofs to living walls to that vase of pampas grass or dahlias in the corner. Many of the Modernist architects of the 1950s and '60s in places like Arizona and California were interested in health and well-being and believed that bringing the outdoors in through walls of glass, inner courtyards, sunrooms, and atriums was key to contentment. They often replaced solid walls, borrowing from Japanese landscape architecture by incorporating light-filtering plants such as bamboo and using brise-soleils (literally "break the sun") such as patterned brickwork and screens that did not block light completely. They had the intuitive feeling that exposure to nature and light was good for our mental health and overall well-being and made a home relaxing and soothing. And now science is beginning to bear that out.

Ecotherapy is a growing scientific field of research dedicated to making connections between the amount of time one spends in nature and levels of depression, stress, and anxiety. In particular, a 2015 study[3] compared two groups that walked for ninety minutes, one in nature and the other in an urban setting. The nature group showed less activity in the frontal cortex of the brain after their walk, which isn't as negative as it might sound. This part of the brain is responsible for "rumination," or repetitive mind chatter around negative emotions. So, it was discovered, walking in nature reduced rumination.

Researchers also believe that having the beauty of nature to look at distracts us from focusing on negative thoughts. This doesn't mean we need to climb a mountain every morning to look at the view. According to a 2016 study published in *Nature Scientific Reports*, when people spent just thirty minutes in parks per week, cases of depression were reduced by 7 percent and cases of high blood pressure by 9 percent.[4] A study of college-age students at Cornell University in 2020 went as far as to say that just ten minutes in a natural environment (even a grassy quad) could improve mood, focus, and physiological markers such as heart rate and blood pressure, and encouraged university designers to incorporate green spaces into their architectural plans.[5]

With technology constantly distracting us, nature takes on an even greater role by alleviating stress and bringing our attention to the ordinary beauty around us. When we stare closely at screens (for an average of four hours a day in North America),[6] altering our depth of field by looking at a sunset on the horizon or an ocean or a mountain can only have a therapeutic effect. It relieves the physical problems that screen time can cause (tech neck is a real thing; ask any chiropractor). And it restores balance, calmness, and let's face it, sanity in the face of all the bad news, cyberbullying, and doom we encounter online.

Nature pulls us up when we feel down, worked up, and vulnerable. It takes us out of our neurosis, shakes off the cobwebs, and helps us to mentally refresh. Nature shows us the way of the cycles and impermanence of all things and awakens the heart.

Forest Bathing

While "forest bathing" has become a trendy practice in the health and wellness community, its roots are in ancient Japanese wisdom. The concept of *shinrin-yoku*—or spending slow, contemplative time in nature—has been around for centuries. This is not about pounding out a trail run at 6 a.m.: it is intentional time to spend walking, observing the light in the trees, listening to the birds, water, wind. It is feeling the air, touching moss, smelling the forest floor, sitting on a log blown down by the wind, or picking up a river rock and holding it in your hand. It is different than just being in nature. It's more like being *with* nature, acknowledging that we, too, are nature. It is in us and it is around us.

Walking in nature does more than promote calm and ease anxiety; it also helps our cognitive functions. When we remove the static and startling noise of technology, industry, and transportation, we suddenly hear better and our intuitive intelligence has a chance to have a voice. Maybe that's why we have our best ideas in the shower? It's like standing under a waterfall. Even more, research has shown that walking in uneven terrain, where we are navigating dips and rises, maybe stepping over branches or streams, has a positive impact on brain function and can even help in recovery from brain injuries, such as strokes.[7] Each step in nature is a small but significant decision: Shall I step over that rock or around it? Walk around that tree or through that puddle? Perhaps that's why mountain climbers are so obsessive about their sport or mushroom foragers so calm and collected—it simply feels good to be immersed in the natural world and be purely focused on present time.

One of my favorite meditation retreat centers is in Onalaska, Washington. It's situated on fifty acres, and the open fields and lush forest provide an ideal location to step away from our programmed ways of living and challenge ourselves in practice. After the first day, we enter into silence and focus inward. Whenever I am there, on my daily walks I can't help but notice the ways the other participants relate deeply to the nature around us. They seem in awe, some gazing in wonder at the horizon or the birds in the sky, others collecting branches to create natural sculptures, and others seemingly just being in the oneness. In their day-to-day lives, some of them teach at universities, manage tech companies, publish prolifically (one very soft-spoken woman had written twelve books in just under a decade). And yet in Onalaska, all of us drop our roles and our attachment to being busy. We find unlimited joy in nature.

Even more amazing is the response of nature to our quiet movement. Just as we open to nature, nature opens to us. During one retreat, a family of deer came around each morning to feast on the fresh grasses. Instead of startling at the sight of humans on the walking path, they relaxed into the moment and watched in interest. Every ten days, another set of eighty meditators infiltrates the deer's home and yet they seemed completely unfazed. They show us the way of trust and curiosity and a way back to our natural human compassion and wisdom.

Finding True Self in Nature

TIME NEEDED: 10 MINUTES

THIS BEAUTIFUL MEDITATION is designed to help root you in the body while affirming the essence of your being. It directs the flow of energy throughout the body, balancing and activating your life force. It's deeply restorative, expanding both your connection with the healing capacity of our earth and the guiding force of the universe.

Let's start by tuning in to the present with intention.

Turn inward by closing your eyes and begin to listen to the breath, the body, and the heart.

Claim the stillness for yourself and rest for a moment.

Feel the body dropping in.

Abandon the endless list of tasks left undone.

And soften your effort.

Now come home to your inner radiance. Be aware of yourself as light illuminating from within, its warmth awakening you.

As you illuminate, notice now a stream of light flowing down from the inner vision of your mind, down the spine, down the leg channels, through the bottoms of the feet, and connecting now to the earth. It's like dropping roots into the rich soil of the earth. Allow anything that doesn't serve to fall away, releasing it to the earth to be transformed into something enriching.

The essence of soul energy is boundless, unrestricted. As this infinite energy moves deeply into the core of the earth, notice the healing support of earth's energy returning nutrients to you. Like a mother who understands her child's needs, she begins to send a healing flow of energy up the legs and into the pelvis, nourishing you.

Know that through earth energy you have an access point to release and transform all that is blocked and all that no longer serves.

Ask the true self to be the guardian of this energy flow.

Now begin to draw your attention to the gateway at the top of the crown.

And invite that gateway to open wide. Feel the healing energy of the sun, the universe, and beyond as it flows downward through the column of the spine. Let it swirl and pool in the pelvis, merging with the rich healing nutrients of earth energy.

Notice now the combined healing energy as it enlivens and expands your life force. Direct it to begin flowing up, through the chest, through the arm channels, up and out of the palms of the hands, releasing anything that may be interfering with your ability to create and manifest the fullest expression of your gifts. Allow another stream to flow from the pelvis up the front body and out through the front of the throat, releasing any blocks to speaking what is true for you. Now take another stream from the pelvis, up the front body, releasing up and out through the crown, clearing anything that may interfere with higher knowing.

Receive now this healing from earth's source and the guiding force of the universe itself. This current of healing is here for your highest good.

With each breath, bring your awareness to that bright and shining light in the inner vision of the mind. Allow that light to expand with a great and unwavering love. With this next exhale, expand that beautiful essence so that it may transcend the body, radiating all around the body and shining far and wide: radiant, brilliant, luminous, and rooted in innate goodness. This is the perfect truth of who you already are. The perfect truth of why you are here.

Breathe, notice, and be.

Artemis's Story: Afterword

The modern Artemis is seen in the woman who refuses to follow the cultural narrative; she loves but can never be claimed. To attempt to control her is to risk losing her altogether. If Artemis takes a partner, they walk beside her, knowing full well that she sees that which is wrong and needs to make it right. She sees all women as her sisters and refuses to join in the harmful gossip that divides us.

Artemis teaches us to stop working on ourselves and to BE ourselves. She seeks an inner balance and knows that to do this well requires the time and space to be with the whispers of the trees and the rivers and creatures of the forest. If you close yourself off from the noise and sit in stillness long enough, you can hear her within yourself.

Top 3 Takeaways

1. To separate ourselves from nature is to remain in suffering. To see ourselves as its essence is to be free.

2. Nature is a source of healing, helping the nervous system to recalibrate and strengthen.

3. When we are separated from the moment, we are separated from ourselves. Nature is a potent way to come back to the present, fully available to the beauty and richness of life.

Journal Prompts

- In what ways are you connecting with your inner Artemis, strong, wise, and an expression of nature itself? What is Artemis teaching you?

- In ancient civilizations, trees were channels for gods and forests were considered temples. How might your life be different if nature became your daily sanctuary?

- What barriers (weather, time commitments) are affecting how you are able to enjoy nature? What if, on the days you aren't able to be in nature, you looked out your window or pictured nature and attuned yourself to the way a tree or flower looks and moves? How might your life be different if you extended your circle of compassion to embrace the whole of nature including yourself?

10

Oneness

Connection and Compassion

*"Oneness is the source of love. Real love is the
One celebrating itself as two."*

RAM DASS

Celia's Story

Therapy is as much soul work as it is a scientific practice to heal the psyche. And when we open to wider planes of consciousness, we begin to see things that can inspire both curiosity and a deep sense of awe. Here is an example.

I was treating a teenage girl—let's call her Celia—who was in agony over her parents' divorce and the constant conflict they were inciting. Celia had very few friends, was deeply depressed and shut down, and held her pain tightly—she had no interest in talking with a complete stranger. I'd worked with enough teens to know that Celia's silence was her superpower, a way to cope and regain some control in a life that had been turned upside down. The basic pledge of a therapist is to "do no harm" and that includes not trying to force someone to talk when it feels threatening to them. Instead, I approached Celia gently with a tray full of sand and invited her to create a world within the tray using any of the hundreds of miniature objects that line several shelves of my office. These could be twigs, rocks, figurines of people, vehicles, houses, fences, and so on. This creative technique called sand tray therapy was first developed by Carl Jung and the idea is that the diorama someone creates is a blueprint for their psyche, how they see themselves and the world itself. This technique bypasses the conscious mind of words to access a part of the psyche that can be reached only nonverbally.

I gave Celia no further instructions. She returned from the shelves with three objects: a girl, a rock, and an umbrella. She placed the umbrella just out of reach of the girl in the sand and stepped away. While she told me nothing of the girl, who she was, or the narrative of her life in this sand tray world, the image she created said it all: a girl alone in a desert without protection. Although this was a significant breakthrough for a teenager who had not revealed very much thus far in our sessions, it was what happened next that astounded me.

The Power of Connection

Among the many things we are learning from the COVID-19 pandemic is just how pervasive loneliness is and what a heavy toll it takes on those who experience it. Many people in long-term care have shown they would rather place themselves at risk of contracting the virus than be deprived of time with their loved ones. Loneliness is by nature a hidden epidemic, and while it's been on the rise for some years now, the pandemic has exposed its scope and prevalence. If you, too, are feeling the effects of loneliness you're not alone. A 2018 survey by the *Economist* showed that almost one in four Americans sometimes or often feels lonely—and that was well before the pandemic hit in 2020.[1] About one-third of Americans aged forty-five and over admitted it to be a significant problem, and for those who are LGBTQIA+ those rates escalated to 49 percent.[2] So how did we get here? And how do we reclaim the meaningful connections and little moments of tenderness that both heal and teach us?

Long-term isolation is not in our nature. We are social beings who long to connect and relate deeply to one another. Yet over the past fifty years, the number of people living alone in the US has more than doubled. In some American cities, this group comprises 40 percent or even more of the population. But being alone and being lonely are two very different things. As you've probably experienced, you can be utterly alone and yet feel completely at peace and joyful in your own company. At other times you can be surrounded by people chattering away at a party, sharing story after story, or be with a group of close friends and feel emotionally desolate. Many women in long-term committed relationships confide they feel completely alone in that relationship year after year. Others have lived away from their partners for long periods of time and continue to feel deeply connected and fulfilled in their hearts. The root of loneliness isn't always the presence or absence of others; it's often a sense of lacking within ourselves.

Although humans may be interdependent by nature, we also have the capacity to relax into the spaciousness of being alone. And while the egoic mind may get caught up in the entangled feelings of anger or resentment or self-pity, loneliness brings our fear patterns front and center. People who feel persistent loneliness are more vulnerable to blaming their feelings on others. They're more at risk of ruminating about how they perceive they are unsupported and unloved, and this tendency compounds a negative feedback loop that leaves them in a cycle of pessimism—and ultimately feeling more alone.[3] When we bring love, compassion, and equanimity into our lives, we no longer see loneliness as a threat. We learn to open to the feelings of loneliness, observe them, and use them to become more compassionate with ourselves. By confronting the inner voice telling us that we're not enough or that we're not worthy on our own, we learn to make peace with loneliness and stop running. We no longer plan and fill our lives with unnecessary activity or crave security through others, and we loosen our grip and attempts to control. Ironically, this positivity is radiantly attractive to others and draws them toward us.[4]

Strengthening Connections

If you were to ask yourself what qualities you most seek in a partner or close friend, funny or adventurous or intelligent might be among the first three to come to mind. And while those are certainly appealing qualities, what many—I'd go so far as to claim most—of us really want is to feel valued and loved. We want someone loving and appreciative, whose heart will truly know us. And even when we understand that true and enduring fulfillment comes only from within, there is nothing like a close relationship to create an emotional landscape that will challenge us and take us into growth. But for love to be truly felt, we need two things: presence and compassion. And to develop those, we need to practice. It may seem hard to believe that sitting and focusing the mind on what we appreciate about a partner or loved one can help cut through life's difficult moments, but neuroscience researchers have found that practicing loving thoughts has a whole lot of merit. In fact, it has the potential to elevate any relationship into a far more loving and connected version—and who wouldn't like that?

Science has caught up to what wisdom teachers have known all along: compassion heals relationships. It strengthens feelings of connection and empathy and infuses a relationship with kindness (even when your partner leaves their socks on the floor—again! or your closest friend ditches your long-awaited dinner plans).[5] Harmonizing the heart and mind in compassionate awareness activates the pleasure circuits in the brain, leaving us feeling deeply content. Add gratitude to the mix, and it's like a booster shot for any relationship, increasing feelings of connection and fulfillment.

Meditation also teaches us to tolerate difficult emotions so that we can more easily turn toward our loved one instead of away. It gives us the practice space to regulate reactivity during painful times and to open empathically to the vulnerability of the moment, making us more available to whatever may be arising.

Invitation to Practice: 20-Second Habits for Strengthening Connection

I'm not usually one for life hacks (transformational growth isn't meant to be a quick fix), but some practices are so immediately beneficial to any relationship they can't be ignored. The following three practices take less than twenty seconds and each is a potent tool for strengthening your connection. Cumulatively, these moments of loving awareness can build trust and a sense of being held in one another's hearts.

TREAT EACH INTERACTION LIKE IT'S THE FIRST ONE

What's the first thing you do when your partner steps through the door? Do you hand over the kids and retreat? Do you throw them a quick glance before you go back to finishing your email? Do you immediately start giving orders on what you need from them? (Yup, I've been there.) And what is the first thing you do when you see a close friend? Do you continue to text? Do you go into an extended rant about the trials and tribulations of your day?

What if, instead, you saw them through fresh eyes? What if you abandoned everything you think you know about your partner or friend and became genuinely curious? Our loved ones are the people to grow and transform with, to love during painful times, and to learn forgiveness through. Love is strongest when it's affirmed through presence. Imagine the impact if you paused more often and gave fuller attention to those in your life. It's often the small things that communicate love most strongly: offering a smile or embrace when a loved one walks through the door after work, thanking them for quietly doing your chores when your back was turned, surprising them with a favorite treat when you know they've had a tough week, putting down your phone when they want to talk.

THE 20-SECOND HUG

Back in the day when our standards for the treatment of animals in research were abysmal, psychologist Harry Harlow carried out a study with infant rhesus monkeys. It went something like this. He took the infants away from their biological mother and gave them two surrogate mothers, one made of wire mesh and another made of terry cloth. Harlow placed the monkeys in one of two conditions. In the first, the wire mesh mother had a bottle for nourishment and the terry cloth mother had no bottle. In the second, the terry cloth mother had the bottle and the wire mesh mother had none. It turns out the baby monkeys spent far more time with the terry cloth mother in both conditions, forgoing food for the feeling of affection. The conclusion was that the baby monkeys would rather starve than let go of their soothing surrogate.[6]

In our touch-deprived culture, we're not unlike Harlow's baby monkeys. Being hugged, and hugged often, doesn't just leave us feeling more connected and loved by our partner and those we're closest to, it's essential for our health. Hugging triggers the brain to release oxytocin (the cuddle hormone that has a big role in the onset of labor), and as it permeates the body it leaves us feeling happier and less stressed. Our blood pressure and heart rate will lower, stress chemicals will plummet, and so too will pain (both emotional and physical). So hug often, hug firm, and hug long (a good twenty seconds to trigger the release of oxytocin).[7] A hug given at the right moment is medicine.

THE 6-SECOND KISS

I've spoken with couples who've healed deep fractures in their relationship and rekindled their connection with the power of the six-second kiss. While it's not a comprehensive solution for the complexities most couples face, it's amazing to see the way it pierces our armor. Kissing releases a chemical cocktail into the blood, starting with oxytocin, that makes us feel safe, close, and connected. Kissing also releases dopamine, the chemical of pleasure that motivates us

As you look at yourself with naked honesty, it can bring up feelings of deep vulnerability. There are no sidetracks or exits in this work, and you're essentially deconstructing the patterns you've based your identity on. You may find yourself challenging how you occupy your time. What you find meaningful may shift. And you may even notice changes in your relationships. As you move from acting in ways you feel you "should" to ways that are true to you, what those around you see might be very different than what they have come to expect. It can feel like a big and daring step to put aside the expectations of our culture or society and learn to stand on our own two feet. Finding other women to share in this work, speak the same language, and lean into when you're exhausted or overwhelmed can be a relief beyond measure. So keep bringing yourself back to your practice, share the dharma of your discoveries, and know that you are not alone. We are all one beating heart.

to seek rewards. Next are epinephrine and norepinephrine, which quicken our heartbeat and leave us feeling like we have butterflies fluttering in our stomach. Finally, kissing reduces cortisol levels, lowering blood pressure and dissolving feelings of stress. All of that can happen in just seconds.

Kissing makes us feel better, brings people closer, and smooths over the rough patches with our partner.[8] But not all kisses are created equal. The kisses with the most impact last at least six seconds. Researcher Dr. John Gottman calls it a kiss with potential. It's a kiss worth coming home to.[9]

The Healing Power of Compassion

I consider compassion to be a human superpower. It gives us the heart intelligence to have genuine concern for others and their well-being—it unifies, heals, and transforms us unlike anything else. Without compassion we are lost in a sea of fear and insecurity, and our ability to trust in humanity dries up. We have now reached a point where the divisions on our planet threaten our physical, social, and emotional well-being. The dedicated practice of compassion has become urgent to end racism, war, climate change, and the many other practices of aggression that divide us. But compassion begins with finding love in ourselves, coming back to our own good heart, and using that love to develop our compassion for others.

If we were to ask all of the women I've worked with over the years what negative beliefs they carry about themselves, one statement would come up more than any other: "I am not enough." In fact, some reports suggest up to 80 percent of women feel this way.[10] And when we internalize this belief, over time it walls us off from the spirit of our true essence and those we long to feel connected to. Feelings of unworthiness fuel the egoic mind, which leads us to compare and prove ourselves to others, strive against them, and ultimately disconnect from the caring that's all around us. Feeling "not enough" seems to be universal for women, despite all the tasks we accomplish each day. If we are to reject the harsh messages of self-criticism and allow love to come and go freely within ourselves, we have to do something that many of us will find challenging in itself: we have to *practice* self-compassion.

Tara Brach—a renowned psychologist, Buddhist teacher, and colleague of mine—said, "Awakening self-compassion is often the greatest challenge people face on the spiritual path."[11] Self-compassion is an ultimate state of self-acceptance. It's a radical act of seeing our true self as human goodness. As we become aware of our true self, we feel more accepting and awakened to the idea that what truly matters lives beyond the physical body, the achievements, notability, and other external trappings of "success." We're talking about authentically and unapologetically allowing ourselves to be human, the slipups, messes, and shadowy moments included. With self-compassion, we disarm judgment with equanimity.

Compassion training recognizes our true interconnectedness: that when one hurts, we all hurt. It is imbued with the desire to actively free others from suffering, and unlike empathy it isn't passive. Paul Bloom, a psychology professor at Yale University, explains that whereas empathy allows us to pick up on and attune to the emotions of others, compassion gives those struggles great weight and impels us to actively try to help. Although what others are feeling may not resonate emotionally with us, we open our heart and mind and value our kinship with them.[12] The distinction is important, because fostering compassion allows us to understand deeply the unifying truth of human suffering and open to the pain with loving kindness. It allows us to actively thwart greed and anger and hate with steadiness, and the impact is far greater than with empathy alone. Compassion brings kindheartedness to the situation, connecting us with what's difficult and dissolving the harm of indifference. True compassion and love have no territorial bounds—they are unconditionally and freely offered through an open and fearless heart.

It feels good to soften into kindness. People who meditate in loving kindness tend to have long-standing happiness that can come only with having an open heart and understanding that a self-focused life is not the way to fulfillment. According to Daniel Goleman, one of the leading researchers in meditation, as little as two weeks of compassion-focused meditation can strengthen the part of the brain that bolsters compassion (including loving kindness for yourself) and empathy, and that same region leaves us feeling happy for doing so.[13] The point is that we're not stuck at one emotional set point. Neuroplasticity means even novice meditators can create changes in their brain system (and most importantly emotional connection) in a matter of weeks.

The question is, How does one generate compassion toward those who have inflicted harm? First of all, we have to accept that we have all harmed. We have all caused pain through patterns of hatred, ignorance, and greed. When we shine the light on our own unwhole-some qualities, we often find ourselves stepping off our high horse and acknowledging that we're not so far removed from those we've judged and condemned.

The Seventeenth Karmapa, a great Buddhist teacher and a com-mitted feminist, once said that when we can no longer bear the suffering of sentient beings, even those that have harmed us, we unleash our full potential to help others and ourselves.[14] To take that first step, we can turn to the wisdom of Tonglen meditation. Tonglen is a Buddhist compassion meditation that literally means "to take" and "to give" in the Tibetan language. It's a tender way to relieve our collective pain and suffering and send peace and well-being to all. It's an approach I learned from Pema Chödrön, the much-loved American Buddhist teacher residing in Gampo Abbey in Nova Scotia. It's a practice I'm dedicated to daily. With Tonglen, we compassion-ately open to the reality of human suffering, softening and educating our hearts while sending out vast healing and relief to ourselves and all others.

I wish the healing practice of Tonglen was taught to the budding hearts and minds of children in grade school everywhere. Imagine the ease it would deliver to children if they learned to hold their experience when they first began to navigate strong emotions. How might their lives be different if they were taught that it's OK to feel vulnerable and that breathing with compassion could support them through the emotional storm? How might our lives have been dif-ferent had we, too, been gently shown that instead of blocking our feelings during moments of pain we can open to our own good heart instead?

Find a quiet, comfortable spot where you can relax into this moment and let's practice together.

Tonglen Meditation
(for Relieving Suffering)

TIME NEEDED: 8 MINUTES

IN THIS MEDITATION we'll soften into compassion, soothe our hearts, and send a current of relief to ourselves and all beings.

Turn inward by closing your eyes or resting the gaze down and ahead of you.

Bring yourself into this moment of quiet stillness.

In slowing down, you can now feel that which has been there all along.

Soften into the heart center and begin to greet yourself with a sense of kindness.

Notice the inner sensations. Be with the breath.

Place a hand at the heart and let the heart be tender.

You might sense the breath lifting you from the weight of your worries.

It's time to remember now, the places where the hurt and the fear and the anger reside.

It's time to let the light shine into the cold and dark places within.

For in this brave act of meeting the pain, we may transform the sorrow.

Notice now any strong emotions you've been facing.

Breathe in fully and draw in the desire to be free from suffering.

Breathe out relief.

Again, breathe in with the desire to be free from suffering.

Breathe out relief.

Take respite in this moment of loving awareness.

Be still and let the breath free each burden and guide you into peace.

Breathe in with the desire to be free from suffering.

Breathe out relief.

Release the pressure from the chest and feel the doors open to the heart.

Remember now your inherent connection with this planet and every being that calls it home.

May we now let the heart govern and guide us toward a more loving path.

Bring to mind those who, too, feel pushed against the torrent of emotion.

Hearts made heavy by the forces of grief, of illness, of fear.

Picture clearly the eyes of those who also need comfort and compassion.

Let the breath trace the pathway from your loving heart to theirs.

Breathe in with the desire to take away their suffering.

Breathe out relief.

Here we use the power of our tenderness to meet the pain together.

Let the heart be soft and filled with ease.

Breathe in with the desire to take away their suffering.

Breathe out relief.

Through each breath, let us heal together with wishes of infinite well-being.

For in this place we bring light to dark waters and surface the truth of our love.

May we dedicate ourselves to relieving the broken hearts of all beings through our words, our actions, and through the alchemy that is our compassion. May we lean in and listen hard. May we speak what is true, especially for those who cannot. May we destroy the illusion of separateness. May we be an unwavering carrier of respect and compassion. And may we heal together.

Breathe, notice, and be.

Self-Forgiveness

Self-forgiveness is about learning to love and forgive ourselves unconditionally. In some ways, it's the ultimate act of self-love: as we make peace with our own heart, we awaken from our trance of unworthiness and hold ourselves with greater compassion. If we can learn the practice of self-forgiveness, we can begin to see our missteps as opportunities for growth and learning rather than as confirmation of our unworthiness. Until we forgive, whether it's ourselves or other people, we run the risk of remaining mired in the past and missing out on the unlimited possibilities of the moment.

Forgiveness is liberating and it is a conscious choice. It is also one of the most potent healing agents we have available to strengthen our body, heart, and mind. Free your heart and you will return to your highest well-being.

7 HEALTH BENEFITS OF FORGIVENESS[15]

1. improves sleep[16]

2. lowers the risk of a heart attack[17]

3. improves cholesterol levels[18]

4. reduces anxiety[19]

5. reduces chronic pain[20]

6. lowers blood pressure[21]

7. mitigates stress[22]

MEDITATION

Ho'oponopono
(for Self-Love and Forgiveness)

TIME NEEDED: 16 MINUTES

HAWAII HAS A long-standing cultural focus on the power of forgiveness. Pu'uhonua o Honaunau is a spiritual sanctuary that has served for centuries as a place of refuge and forgiveness. In ancient Hawaii, those who committed wrongdoing and reached this site would be pardoned and sent home with a newly birthed commitment to making their body the temple of forgiveness. Ho'oponopono meditation is an extension of the Hawaiian people's fortitude for forgiveness. It means "to make it right." In this practice, you'll recite a four-verse mantra and direct its message to your own heart: "I'm sorry. Please forgive me. I love you. I thank you."

The version of Ho'oponopono below focuses on self-forgiveness and self-love, two qualities that most of us lack. Women tend to support and nourish the needs of others while depriving ourselves of the kind of self-appreciation and honoring needed to feel whole and worthy. This practice may feel odd and uncomfortable at first. Your unconscious mind patterns may try to hold you in the current of insecurity and shame. But in time, repeating the mantra will set you on track to a gentler, kinder, and more loving way. Self-compassion is our most reliable source of inner strength.

Let's begin.

Turn inward by closing your eyes and place the hand at the heart for a moment.

Feel now your authentic presence.

Begin to settle the heart and calm the mind through the simple practice of breath awareness.

As you breathe through the nose, just allow the natural inhale to fill the lungs, and then release any tension through a natural exhale.

Troubled times will continue to unfold in life, but through practice you can begin to meet those difficulties with greater kindness. What you give your time and attention to now becomes your lived embodiment later. Take a moment to give yourself permission to commit fully to this practice of self-compassion.

May this Ho'oponopono meditation be your chapel of self-honoring.

May this be a time of intentional healing.

May you open fully to the practice of apologizing, forgiving, loving, and appreciating yourself.

Let the breath take you more deeply inward to those places of holding, the storerooms of hurt and pain. Look now at all those times you have been hard on yourself or held yourself in judgment or told yourself that you're not enough.

Take a deep, slow breath in and open the heart. Repeat these words inwardly:

I'm sorry.
Please forgive me.
I love you.
I thank you.

Notice the response of the body as it takes in this healing message. Let the words permeate through your entire being.

Bring to mind all the times you criticized your physical appearance, denied your hunger, deprived yourself of sustenance because you believed you had not earned it, or overworked your body because you felt you weren't enough. Notice the ways you've held yourself to an unreasonable and harmful standard.

Take a deep, slow breath in and feel the heart opening to receive these words.

I'm sorry.
Please forgive me.
I love you.
I thank you.

Feel into this message of healing and forgiveness. Release whatever shame or self-judgment may be ready to clear and allow it to ground through the earth.

Bring to mind all the times you missed an opportunity because you doubted yourself or felt small, or because you were told it was wrong to want it.

Take a deep, slow breath in.

I'm sorry.

Please forgive me.

I love you.

I thank you.

For any times you didn't honor yourself with healthy boundaries or you stayed in relationships that harmed you or did not align with the current of your life because you were afraid to leave. For all the times you turned your back on yourself and failed to be the friend you so badly needed, take a deep, slow breath in.

I'm sorry.

Please forgive me.

I love you.

I thank you.

For all of the times you took on the judgment and blame of others because you felt powerless, and for any time you fell into self-sabotaging behavior or harmed yourself, take a deep, slow breath in.

I'm sorry.

Please forgive me.

I love you.

I thank you.

For all the times you knew your words would hurt but you said them anyway, take a deep, slow breath in.

I'm sorry.

Please forgive me.

I love you.

I thank you.

Let every breath wash away the unconscious patterns of disdain, and let the heart bring new waves of compassion to soothe the pain that set in the shadows. Take a deep, slow breath in.

I'm sorry.
Please forgive me.
I love you.
I thank you.

Feel now the inflow of healing light moving down through the crown and into the column of the body, releasing any blocks to your highest well-being. For all those times you were swept into the undercurrent of fear and were lost in harmful thoughts, take a deep, slow breath in.

I'm sorry.
Please forgive me.
I love you.
I thank you.

Know that you did the best that you could at the time. Sink into the heart center and begin to feel yourself renewed by the healing force of your own heart. Let the heartbeat sound like a beacon to the rest of the body, as if to remind you that you are whole, have always been whole. Anchor into this mantra as the energy within your cells, tissues, and organs expands beyond the physical body to be one with everything around you. For all those times you saw yourself as separate and allowed the small self to reign sovereign, take a deep, slow breath in.

I'm sorry.
Please forgive me.
I love you.
I thank you.

Feel the deep sense of forgiveness and compassion expanding from the heart. For all the times that you stepped outside of the doorway of the heart and forgot the truth of your innate goodness, take a deep, slow breath in.

I'm sorry.
Please forgive me.

I love you.

I thank you.

May we all find forgiveness in the shadows of anger, choose love over hatred, and release our hearts from resentment. Let the body, mind, and spirit receive fully the grace of love and forgiveness and remember there is only radiance here. Take a deep, slow breath in.

May we all embody the spirit of loving kindness and may we be at peace.

Breathe, notice, and be.

Celia's Story: Afterword

When Celia's session with the sand tray was over, she left and I returned the objects to their places on the shelves. Three hours later, another client arrived for her session. She was older, her life story was completely different from Celia's, and she and Celia had never met. When I suggested she create a sand tray world, she chose the same three objects that Celia had and placed them in the exact same positions in the tray. I was stunned. Was she picking up on Celia's unconscious energy transmuted to the same three objects and still detectable three hours later? Or was she picking up on communication from a shared consciousness? Or was something else guiding her to the same three objects out of several hundred? I'll never know, but what I do know is that as humans we are deeply interconnected. And when we honor and foster that connection, it can be healing beyond measure.

Top 3 Takeaways

1. Our relationships are an invitation to do the gritty work of self-realization. Every relationship is an opportunity to become more present and compassionate.

2. True compassion and love have no territorial bounds—our life is a training ground to offer them and receive them freely.

3. Authentic forgiveness is a potent healing agent; it brings heart and mind together in an unobstructed love.

Journal Prompts

- Sometimes the act of describing the feelings behind loneliness can minimize its emotional bite. What does loneliness feel like for you? Describe and get to know the emotions, sensations, thoughts, and behaviors that arise when you're feeling lonely. What would it be like to open to those feelings fully and confront the fear with compassion?

- What does support and connection mean to you? Is there an outpouring of love that you're unable to give and receive at this time in your life? What small step could you take today to change that?

- What in your life do you wish you could forgive yourself for? What feelings arise as you think about this experience?

- Write a letter of forgiveness to yourself to release all that you've been holding. Include what you've learned and the ways those events have created openings for growth.

11

Ritual and Creativity

Expressing the True Self

"You can't use up creativity.
The more you use, the more you have."

MAYA ANGELOU

Karyn's Story

"Let's check in with your body. Now begin to scan and notice where you feel that sense of peace you've been talking about. You might close your eyes if that feels OK and just see where you can make contact with that feeling of inner calm. Don't worry if you can't sense it right away; just trust that it's there."

As I offered these words, Karyn began to find a peacefulness she had forgotten existed within her. She sighed deeply and visibly began to relax into her body. I encouraged her to send the breath into the places of tension and to place her hands on her heart and belly to connect more deeply with the emotional truth that resided there. I invited her to let her mind travel all the way back to one of the first times she'd ever felt those sensations. "It was so long ago," she said as tears began to roll down her cheeks. She was revisiting a time unbound by the emotional stress and hurt of a relationship that had swept her feet out from right under her.

I'd met Karyn shortly after she'd moved across the country to protect herself from an abusive relationship she'd endured for years. Andy (her ex-boyfriend) was a childhood friend whose familiar friendship made him a safe bet for a first boyfriend—at least on paper. But as the intensity of the relationship grew over time, so did Andy's anger. During an earlier session, she'd shared, "I felt so sorry for him. I thought that if I just stayed with him it would get better. When things were good, they were really good—he was so loving and funny. And I didn't want to abandon him. He just seemed to need me so much and he always promised he'd work on himself. In truth, I didn't want to lose him, and no one said anything—not even his parents—when they heard him screaming at me in the next room. I was told that Andy had always been a hothead and that I should just step out of the room when he was raging; it became my responsibility to be more understanding and to manage him somehow." As in most cycles of abuse, Andy's feelings of jealousy and reactivity mounted over time. The couple became more isolated and insular: the traumatic patterns of aggression followed by attempts to repair the hurt were mostly hidden, and what was witnessed was largely ignored. Karyn was brave beyond measure to have left an entire life behind to save her own.

As she kept breathing and settled into her body, she began to bring forward earlier times of inner calm. "I'm thinking about elementary school, before I knew Andy. I was so innocent," she said. "I can remember spending hours and hours on my artwork: painting and drawing and pasting together a mosaic of stones and leaves and whatever moved me. I didn't question whether it was beautiful or worthy or time well spent. I didn't care if other people liked it or saw me as talented. I created for myself." Those memories of creating artwork were enlivening a connection with a forgotten part of herself, and the more Karyn spoke, the more joyful she became. She paused suddenly and her eyes widened. "I think this is the way back to myself: I need to start creating again."

Transforming Our Life with Ritual

Ritual is one of the earliest languages of healing. Dance, rhythm, drumming, chanting, altars, and symbols have traditionally made up the lexicon that transcends the egoic mind and opens us to our inner essence. Ritual makes sacred what may seem ordinary, brings a freshness to the present, and reminds us that in every moment we can be made anew. Through ritual we are never lost; instead, we linger in the liminal space of infinite possibility. The rituals and routines we commit to hold the space for transformation. And when we take time to reflect inwardly, and purposefully shape our day in ways that cultivate appreciation, awe, and wonder, we transform the quality of our entire life.

When practiced consistently, restorative rituals have widely positive effects on mental health and emotional well-being.[1] Each small step adds up to radical changes in our health, outlook, mood, and neurobiology. Yet many of the women I work with keep their rituals well hidden. They worry that their practices of self-honoring will be seen by others as silly, superstitious, or indulgent or that they'll be judged for spending time that could be better devoted to ticking off more items on the to-do list. They "sneak in" the practices that amplify their very essence and provide an important bridge between their inner and outer worlds. By design, rituals are reliable and help us to connect deeply to the sacred in ourselves and everything before us.

The rituals that you build your life around will be deeply personal: they may be formed through your cultural heritage, spiritual beliefs, or family traditions. Routines and rituals require active participation: they thrive in mindful awareness and dedicated intention. So not only do morning rituals, daily walks in nature, afternoon tea, prayer, and daily stretching calm the nervous system, they also shape our life. Remember, the scientific dharma tells us that whatever we repeat we become. So whatever rituals you choose, check in and ask, "Does this soothe my soul?"

Invitation to Practice: Calling in Sacred Ritual

Ritual, the repetition of action we relax into, can soothe and restore, energize and strengthen. Through ritual we slow down, open, and give the mind and body the spaciousness they crave. Ritual invites us into the present moment in its fullest possibility.

Dream now of the routines and rituals that form your life. What do you practice in secret or yearn to call into each day? A poem whispered softly? A lit candle? Soft music carrying you through the morning light? Writing in the pages of a journal? A warm salt bath on Sunday night? Dancing alone? A cold plunge in the dark waters of a lake? Letters of gratitude? The smell of freshly baked bread? The fresh scent of a cut blossom? A chapter read? Each of these rituals may not be enough to notice at first, but in time they all weave the life lived well.

As you sit in quiet contemplation, open to the rhythms that move you, soothe you, and inspire you. Set an intention now to meet this ritual each day and allow it to manifest as a physical expression of your inner essence.

To honor your ritual, repeat this mantra ever so quietly: "I do this in the spirit of healing and awakening."

The Healing Power of Creativity

What if we could weave our well-being or form our inner peace with clay or settle our mind with each stroke of a paintbrush? Thinking ceases when the hands take over, because the mind can only truly focus on one thing at a time. When we write lyrics, plant a garden, cook a meal, throw a pot on a pottery wheel, paint, or sketch, we not only ease the overactive mind; we also give voice to the soul. These are gifts that lie on the other side of awareness, yearning to be seen, shared, and heard.

I recently heard a poignant story about a patient at an all-male addiction treatment center who had learned to knit on a loom in an art therapy class while he was in jail. He found it quelled anxiety and gave him an outlet for his creativity. He continued to knit at the treatment center, and rather than mock him, as one might expect in an all-male environment, his fellow patients took an interest. One by one, they too acquired looms and wool, eventually forming a knitting club. Soon the group had knit enough toques—more than 200—to supply an emergency shelter and a women's addiction treatment center. Next, they set out to knit tiny hats for the newborns at the local children's hospital. When interviewed by the local news outlet, one man said that knitting was like meditating for him, that it took his mind away from his problems. But his favorite part was finishing a toque and giving it away. "It's really nice to start something and finish it,"[2] he said.

Creativity and the heart are like twin sisters, not identical but deeply attuned, each supporting the other in her purpose. We release our anguish on the canvas or over the pages of our journal. Our hands intuitively trace the lines back to our emotional calluses and nodules, applying the balm that allows us to soften into ourselves. In time, we release the shadows inside and rediscover the light.

Many of us are afraid of our creativity. We say things like "I'm not artistic" or "I could never do that." Yet all of us are born with limitless potential. As young children, we are unencumbered by egoic thoughts of who we are and even more, who we are not. Yet as we get older, our openness to possibility narrows and the identities we've adopted begin to shadow the discovery that once came so effortlessly. By the time we are adults, we've been self-limiting for so long that we've lost sight of what is possible. But to create is to express the deepest parts of ourselves, the parts left unnamed, unspoken. To create is to open a portal to a healing we may not have known we needed.

Let me tell you another story. By the time I was thirty-eight years old, I had been a therapist for almost a decade. In therapist years, a decade is considered infancy. Teaching the heart how to heal from pain, grief, violence, and terror takes years of practice. And I was feeling burned out. Sleep didn't come easily, and in truth it wasn't welcome. Each night I was met with the same scene: I would climb a steep mountain, my legs buckling with the weight at my back and sweat pouring from my brow. Clinging to my back were arms and legs, an entanglement of bodies all culminating into one. I was carrying the sorrow and suffering of every client I had ever seen. Each morning I was met with a deep sense of dread. I had recently lost a seventeen-year-old client to a cocaine overdose and was terrified someone else under my care would die.

Finally I went to see a great friend, a colleague and mentor whose steadiness and kindness had helped me countless times before. He knew of the guilt I carried and that the grief I held deep in my bones wasn't just clouding my mind; it was affecting my physical health. He listened patiently and then encouraged me to find a way to release the pain. "Find a way, Michele. Write about it, keep a dream journal, draw, paint, listen to what calls you. Let the unconscious make its way through the pages and the paint and the dreams." When I returned to my office, I pulled out a canvas and some paints I had stored away. I had been working with teens with developmental disabilities and found that art was a potent way for them to express their inner world when words didn't come easily. I took the lid off the paint jar, dipped in the brush, and swept the paint across the canvas trusting my friend's words. I painted and painted, bought larger canvases, and dedicated myself to covering each one. And with each completed canvas, I sensed a release in my body. I began to breathe easier and I entered into the current of healing. After only a few weeks, the nightmares dissolved and the anxiety dissipated. I was restored.

The only thing standing between ourselves and the expression of our many gifts is us. To starve our creativity is to deny our life-giving nature. When we free ourselves to play and craft and dance

In this culture of competition, it's easy for the egoic mind to get trapped in a narrative of "lack." Many women tell me they feel as though they're "falling behind" and that everyone else is achieving, progressing, or somehow doing better than they are. My heart hurts when I see these false beliefs weighing them down and dimming their vibrancy. I invite them to join me in an exercise to reintroduce them to their inner wisdom. I invite you to try it too.

Take a moment to turn inward and settle into the body. And let the mind's eye take you on a journey into the vast wilderness of your inner self. Imagine now that you're walking along a pathway—a velvet mossy trail. Clusters of California poppies are huddled together, bowed in the light drizzle. The mist has erased all sense of time. A light burns its way through the fog and leads you to a sturdy hut with smoke rising from the chimney. The door is ajar, inviting you to take refuge with the wise woman within. Her wisdom has been simmering like a good dense broth. You step inside to meet your much older self. She holds the eye of compassion, a gaze that melts layers around your heart. She welcomes the questions you've longed to have answered, sagacious and loving in her replies. You stay for a while to seek her counsel and open to her guidance. And then as you prepare for your return journey, she takes your hands in hers and says: "Be gentle with yourself, dear one. You're exactly where you are meant to be."

in our artistry, we enliven ourselves and we begin to heal. When we express outwardly, we feed ourselves inwardly, and honor the wild and mysterious forces of mind and heart and spirit all at once. So let us lay hands in clay, pluck melodies with strings, and be made alive through the outpouring of creation.

Illuminating as Light
(Supporting Creative Flow)

TIME NEEDED: 12 MINUTES

THIS MEDITATION WILL support you toward becoming deeply present and expansively aware of the unlimited potential of your creative flow.

When you are ready, turn inward by closing your eyes. Come into quiet stillness. Take in a low, slow breath, and remember there is no better use for time than this today. A time to open the mind and rest in the infinite, where the past is no more and where you exist in the brilliance of your light.

Root in the body, taking a moment now to feel it fully. You might notice the spaciousness in and around the body. Now begin to scan the body from the top of the head, all the way down to the toes, and sense where you feel open or closed to the creative flow. Don't try to change it; just allow yourself to feel it.

Now begin to draw your attention to wherever your awareness meets the breath. Perhaps at the nostril, at the upper lip, or the belly. With each breath, become aware of the movement. The breath is always there, constantly available, faithfully returning you to this moment. It asks only that you notice.

Take some time now to notice the thoughts that may be blocking your fullest expression of creativity. Bring forward the mental obstacle or story you've been telling yourself about your creative capacity. You may think, "I don't have enough time."

Or perhaps, "This has been done before." Or you may wonder, "Am I good enough?" Whatever the thoughts may be, just observe, allow, and witness them with kindness.

Now be aware of a shining light in the inner vision of your mind. That light is the essence of you, the you that you were born as, the embodiment of pure love and infinite goodness. Allow that light to expand until it fully inhabits the body. Let that light permeate through the bones, the organs, the muscles, enlivening every cell of your being.

Notice the inner sensations. Become aware of those areas that you have forgotten, where you have not been fully present. Notice, without judgment, and shine a little brighter there.

With this next exhale, turn up your light, expand your beautiful essence, so that it transcends the body, shining far and wide: radiant, brilliant, luminous, and rooted in innate goodness. This is the perfect truth of who you already are. The perfect truth of why you are here.

Now create a clear fluid boundary all around you at arm's length and let it serve as a beautiful definition of where your essence touches the vast outer field. Outside of that clear fluid boundary, picture a rose. Put whatever may be blocking your creative expression into the rose, and now let it go. No matter what appears, just know it for the moment and then let it fall away. Release it fully.

Put whatever may be blocking you in the rose and let it go a few more times. Simply observe the sensations. You might begin to feel a lightness or an inner spaciousness or the sensations may remain the same. Just allow yourself to be curious and open.

Now reconnect again with your inner light, your core essence, shining from the inner vision of your mind, filling the body, illuminating the skin, and extending all the way out to arm's length. Feel the pure light.

Sink into the heart center and rest deeply in the spaciousness of your beautiful radiance. Now, place a drop of your pure light energy into the clear fluid boundary. Allow it to enliven and charge up your entire being with the strongest current of your creative life force.

Imagine that when you paint, write, draw, craft, weave, put hands in clay, you manifest freely, unapologetically, and above all else, that you create with unwavering compassion toward yourself. Let creativity flow freely from the wellspring of your light.

Breathe, notice, and be.

Move through your day in the fullest expression of your radiance: be as light, knowing that this is the truth of why you are here.

Karyn's Story: Afterword

I am often reminded that within ourselves we have everything we need to grow and heal and transcend our greatest difficulties. This seemed undeniably so with Karyn. While healing the trauma of an abusive relationship through therapy, she rediscovered her core essence—the enduring light of inner self—through creativity. She returned to therapy again and again sharing stories of discovery. She pored over her old sketchbooks, started new ones, painted and glued and pounded clay—everything became a means of self-expression and healing. She naturally incorporated ritual into her practice, collecting crystals and stones and artifacts and placing them throughout her apartment with the confidence of a woman who knows herself well. With every moment of creative expression, Karyn was releasing and metabolizing the pain and terror held deeply in her body. It is an unconscious process of healing available to us all.

Top 3 Takeaways

1. Ritual makes sacred what may seem ordinary and reminds us that in every moment we can be made anew. It roots us in the present and brings a healing rhythm to our lives.

2. Ritual is an invitation to slow down and connect with a wider realm of consciousness. When we do this, we're able to invigorate ourselves, balance our energy, and listen to a vast intelligence available to us always.

3. To create is to express the deepest part of ourselves, the parts left unnamed, unspoken. To create is to open a portal to a healing we may not have known we needed.

Journal Prompts

- Write about a ritual that you can use each day to honor yourself and bridge your inner and outer worlds. It can be as simple as pausing and taking a deep breath before you place your feet on the floor, reciting a mantra, setting an intention, or giving thanks for the day.

- Think back to your childhood. What creative activities did you do? How did you feel while doing them? Write about some of the creative activities you'd like to welcome back into your life.

- Write the story of your creative gifts. Include the narratives you've inherited or held about what it means to be a creative being and the ways you've held back or stopped yourself from expressing yourself fully.

12

Gratitude

Embracing the Everyday

"I don't have to chase extraordinary moments to find happiness—it's right in front of me if I'm paying attention and practicing gratitude."

BRENÉ BROWN

Shona's Story

Shona wasn't a new client. I had seen her through the unimaginable loss of her newborn son, a painful divorce, and more recently two car accidents that had left her in chronic pain. She had approached therapy in much the same way she tackled life itself, with fierce courage. For months she had battled with sleeplessness and an overwhelming sense of dread. She was newly remarried, and conversations had begun about starting a family. She couldn't shake the thought that her body might betray her, that she was somehow broken, and that life was merciless. She carried a deep resentment for the mistakes made by the doctors during the delivery of her baby,

215

the ways her ex-husband had withdrawn and abandoned her in her grief, and worse yet, she blamed herself for almost everything that had happened since.

I've come to see my clients not as people needing to be cured, but as wise beings who are teaching as much as they are transforming. Shona was no different. We talked with raw vulnerability about the past. She discovered ways to open to the most painful of feelings and talked to her younger self with great compassion, soothing and reassuring her and reminding her of her strength. She reflected on the many women who had come before who'd also experienced heartbreaking loss and on the power she was finding in sharing her story through her music and her writing. And most recently, she had discovered the grace that comes with forgiveness.

Somatic therapy had helped to guide Shona to the unconscious effects of trauma held in her tissues and organs and generated a way to release and remove the trapped pain. We had worked together with breath work; EMDR (eye movement desensitization and reprocessing, a therapeutic technique that helps to release trauma and reintegrate the subconscious); meditation; and eating the right foods to support her physical and emotional healing. She had added healing practices into her lifestyle one by one until she felt renewed. It took time, and there were many shifts and setbacks. But she was her own best healer, repeatedly guiding herself into the unknown with great resiliency.

Shona and I began to explore the symbols in her art, meditations, and dreams. I'm often amazed by the divine symbols that push forward during times of great healing and one of Shona's called our attention: the lotus, one of the most potent images of purity and healing found in the texts of Mahayana Buddhism. While it's rooted and grows in the muck, the lotus blooms as a beautiful white flower. According to myths, lotus flowers bloomed in the steps of the baby Buddha. It symbolizes the sacred enlightenment that is born through the painful experiences in our lives. We remain pure, despite all of the suffering.

I asked, "Do you have a sense of why this symbol is showing itself to you now?"

The Power of Gratitude

Do you remember how often your mother told you to be grateful? Whether her motives were about shaping behavior and personality or educating the heart and mind, the science behind her advice was solid. It's a heart habit that is especially potent when we focus on the appreciation we have for our parents or those who have raised us: feeling grateful for those who brought us into the world and nurtured us has been found to dissolve anger,[1] strengthen pathways for happiness,[2] and quash depression.[3] Now imagine the strength of extending that appreciation to everyone you come across in your day.

Gratitude is essentially an appreciation for the basic goodness in all things, and that starts with oneself, especially when it feels difficult to do so. Most women are masters at expressing appreciation, and our innate capacity to attune to the emotions of others primes us to share generously. Our work lies in extending that kindness to ourselves. Have you noticed how often you blame yourself when things don't go as expected or you're overtaken by fear, irritability, and other expressions of inner pain? The anxious mind forgets gratitude because it's constantly scanning the landscape for danger, even if that means turning against the self to enable a false sense of control. But the critical mind seems to dissolve in the warm environment of appreciation. When we take a moment to pause, breathe, and mindfully look at the situation, we begin to see that life is filled with uncomfortable moments and that no one is immune to discomfort or difficulty. Imagine the freedom of letting go of judgment and instead leaning into those difficult moments with relaxed openness and gratitude for your strength and resilience.

The practice of being grateful has gained a lot of attention in both the self-help and neuroscientific community in the past decade, and for good reason. It's deeply healing when we allow ourselves to see the grace and beauty that is found in the ordinary aspects of our lives. While the negativity bias of the critical and anxious mind may resist, training ourselves to stay with the openheartedness of gratitude pays off in spades.[4] How might this world be different if each of us felt contentment for what exists before us? How might our spirit be supported and enlivened if we recognized and paid attention to the gifts and opportunities we already have? When we pause, notice, give ourselves fully to the moment, delight in the sweetness of a cup of tea, a good night's sleep, and the joy of visiting with a friend, the mind and emotions align with the sacred that lies in each day. The magic of integration takes center stage.

Gratitude, when practiced over time

- strengthens the pathways for a positive mind[5]
- lowers stress levels[6]
- improves mental health resiliency[7]
- fosters greater life satisfaction[8]
- bolsters wisdom[9]

Let's take a look at some of the compelling ways in which gratitude turns our heart away from destructive emotions. In Buddhist practice it's believed that three primary emotions (the three poisons) drive our suffering: passion (also called craving or greed), aggression (aversion or anger), and ignorance (indifference). Gratitude dulls the sharp edges and softens the impact of the three poisons, shaping our lives to drop resentment, anger, and other negative emotions that exacerbate our stress levels and destroy our sense of satisfaction and joy (not to mention our relationships). When we embrace gratitude, we feel more connected and naturally begin to take action, repairing those relationships where we have caused harm. It empowers us as agents of change. Writer Melody Beattie summed up gratitude perfectly when she wrote: "Gratitude unlocks the fullness of life. It turns what we have into enough, and more. It turns denial into acceptance, chaos to order, confusion to clarity. It can turn a meal into a feast, a house into a home, a stranger into a friend."[10]

When life gets extra hard it can feel personal and permanent. But no matter how long you've been where you
are, nothing stays the same. Everything in life is moving
through: the seasons, the tides, the plants and animals
and fungi in your garden, and yes, your own human
life is constantly changing (even when it doesn't feel
that way). The Buddhist term for this impermanence is
anicca ('ænikə), and when I feel stuck or caught up in hot
emotions or when I am facing loss I make that word my
mantra. I repeat "Aniccaaaaaa" and I really draw out the
final aaaah sound. When we live with the awareness of
impermanence, everything begins to shift. We realize
there's really no place to get to and so we begin
to relax into our lives with wonder and gratitude.
Give it a try. Anicca.

Our Brain on Gratitude

Let's take a closer look at the ways in which gratitude can activate
our brain, rewiring it for a life rich with openhearted presence and
appreciation. The active choice to stop and intentionally turn the
thinking mind to appreciation leads the brain to release a surge of
neurotransmitters associated with emotional well-being. A single
dose of gratitude can increase both dopamine, which is associated
with pleasure, motivation, and emotional heightening, and serotonin, the happiness neurochemical that stabilizes mood.[11] When
we feel good, our body can naturally counteract any symptoms of
anxiety, depression, and stress.

Research also shows that writing about the things we're most
grateful for activates the ventromedial prefrontal cortex, the area
of the brain responsible for our desire to be altruistic.[12] Activating
this reward center boosts our sense of connection, supporting the
heart-centered wisdom this world so badly needs. Other areas of the

brain that become strengthened when we're grateful are the hypo-thalamus (the body's control center for sleep, hunger, metabolism, and other regulatory mechanisms) and the medial prefrontal cor-tex (learning and decision-making). Research by science researcher Robert A. Emmons and his colleagues has shown that there are multiple physical, psychological, and social benefits to keeping a gratitude journal[13] and that people who practice gratitude are more likely to remember positive information than negative.

His research shows that two elements work together in a heal-ing alchemy: the awareness of goodness and the acknowledgment of the source of that goodness. So, unlike pride, which is inherently self-interested, gratitude is the humble acceptance that goodness exists in all others, even when they're acting in ways that hurt us. As counterintuitive as it may seem, when we begin to see the hurt and anger and the ways others are triggering our karmic baggage as an invitation to grow, gratitude comes to the fore. Gratitude clears our neuroses, soothes the anxious mind, and empowers our ability to say what needs to be said with clarity and compassion.

What's more, Emmons found four ways that practicing gratitude regularly can affect our well-being.

1. Gratitude returns us to the reality of the present, waking us to the poetic beauty of life, right alongside its challenges. It requires active participation. Gratitude is not a passive feeling or fleeting thought; it's an invitation to connect to a sense of awe and wonder, which we cannot do when we're ruminating about the past or predicting the future.

2. Gratitude can educate the heart and mind away from negative emotions, such as fear and regret; it may even ward off depression. Gratitude, it seems, is incompatible with negative feelings: we can't feel both at once. For example, the more grateful we feel, the less envious we are.

3. Gratitude acts as a buffer to stress, and those who practice gratitude recover from trauma more quickly.

4. The lived experience of gratitude leaves us feeling more confident and worthy, which many women tell me they struggle with.

Authentic gratitude is an expression of love for the life before us—all of it. American road cyclist and Olympic gold medalist Kristin Armstrong summed this up beautifully when she said, "When we focus on our gratitude, the tide of disappointment goes out and the tide of love rushes in."

The 8 Sacred Soul Qualities of Gratitude

Practicing gratitude offers so much more than many of us realize. Its soul quality extends beyond the thinking mind and into many other aspects of our lived experience. In fact, researchers have discovered that within gratitude lie eight sacred qualities. This is where we take the practice of gratitude beyond the mental mind-set and into the enduring embodiment of our own nature.

1. **Awe:** A sense of awe emerges as we tap into the sacred connection between ourselves and all that exists before us. The sun setting, the sound of a beautiful voice, the essence of emotion, the brilliance and beauty that lie in nature, the birth of a child—all of these things can leave us moved beyond words. We are speechless in our deep appreciation of the magic in our lives.

2. **Appreciation of the present moment:** Attuning our awareness to the beauty of the present moment is like pointing our internal compass toward the path of open, conscious awareness. Arriving in the present helps us to harmonize our cognition and emotion and connect and appreciate all that exists before us. When we become distracted and find ourselves lost in the mental forest of negative thinking, we tend to feel a lack of agency. But each time we return to the now, we awaken to the potential of the moment.

3. **Internal abundance:** This is a sense of deep knowing that everything we seek already lies within us. It's an awareness that we are already

whole. We are grateful for the health, connection, creativity, nature, spirituality, and abundance within us. And instead of striving to be thinner, more stylish, or more successful, we become attuned to the truth that we have always been enough. And we work toward changing that which no longer serves us in our lives from a place of joy rather than inner lacking.

4. **Compassionate comparison:** The conditioned mind continuously scans, compares, and categorizes endless streams of information. All too often we make ourselves feel better by comparing our circumstances to the misfortune of others (also known as schadenfreude). For example, we hear of a couple separating and feel a little better about our own relationship. Or we learn about a business closing and feel more optimistic about our own financial struggles. We see this pattern in advertisements, music, movies, novels, and just about every social reference point. But it doesn't feel right or good. In contrast, compassionate comparison is healing and supportive to authentic gratitude. In this practice, we hold the suffering of others in our awareness with an eye to how fortunate we are, wishing that same good fortune for them. When we practice this gratitude often enough, we both strengthen and turn our heart and mind toward helping those in need. The compassionate heart isn't complacent but fierce in its convictions.

5. **Appreciation of others:** When a friend reaches out because she sees you withdrawing or a coworker helps you meet a deadline, you undoubtedly feel a deep sense of gratitude and relief in knowing you're seen and valued and in not facing life's struggles alone. The ability to accept and lean into the help and care of others is empowering and can strengthen relationships, but many women have to consciously practice doing this. Many of us feel indebted or guilty when we receive support, but when did you last look down on a female friend who accepted help from you? It's okay to be that friend accepting help.

6. **The wisdom of adversity:** I am constantly in awe of the grace that finds us while we're in even the strongest storms of adversity. There are times when we are so swept up and thrown adrift by the difficulties in life that we wonder how we'll ever find our way back to shore, and we surrender to the current. In time, we return to shore and find ourselves in a place of growth. Adversity is a great teacher. Even during our greatest challenges, a thin ray of light will appear to show us the way to the beauty that is our lives. And after hardship, we often begin to appreciate the things we took for granted that have not been lost and the things that have been gained.

7. **The power of ritual:** Embodied gratitude requires practice. The rituals and routines we commit to are the path of our becoming. Taking time to reflect inwardly and purposefully about what we hold dear will cultivate a consciousness of appreciation and transform our lives.

8. **Oneness:** The suffering of our modern age has emerged in part from a culture that favors individualism over interdependence. What if we began to see the intelligence of our oneness, that when we care for one another, we also contribute to and help heal the greater whole? Each and every time we make appreciation and gratitude a part of our natural language, we transmute its power to others, so they, too, begin to embody loving appreciation.

The Gratitude Journal

Quite often when I'm working with clients, we close a session by activating an intention to practice a tool or make a daily, manageable shift toward greater well-being. It's through the small day-to-day shifts, what I call micro shifts, that radical and bold changes happen. When I run down the menu of the most potent daily practices for transforming our lives, there is one tool above all others that clients are likely to tell me they practice without fail: the gratitude journal.

Emmons, as we saw, is also a strong proponent, and his studies show that keeping a gratitude journal for just three weeks can have a measurable positive effect on psychological well-being and relationships.[14] Spending time each day to reflect on the aspects of our life that we feel deeply grateful for is simple and powerful. The key is being willing to take a few moments to sink into the heart, soften into the moment, and stay there a while. So often we believe that something needs to be difficult for it to be meaningful or worthwhile. Nothing could be farther from the truth. Our lives are built on simple and sacred moments.

Our culture has become so big, so busy, and so loud that we chase the macro moments to confirm that our lives matter. Once we're granted that promotion, we think, or achieve those 10,000 social media followers or move into the next biggest home, *then* we'll look at our lives with appreciation. But we lose touch with the beauty that lies before us, unconditionally and always. Martin Seligman, who is known as the father of positive psychology, leads the way in a field that studies the science of the well-lived life. One of his studies particularly stands out for me and meets the gold standard in terms of scientific rigor (it's randomly assigned and placebo controlled).

Seligman gathered a group of participants and asked them to set aside ten minutes every night for a week. He asked them to write down three things that went well each day and why they went well. The event didn't need to be grand or earth-shattering; it just needed to be acknowledged and recorded.[15] Just as I'd seen with my clients, a significant number of participants in Seligman's study continued to make a ritual of noting what went well every day—even six months after the study ended.[16] They reported feeling less depressed and more enduringly happy in their lives. The daily act of expressing appreciation for life's positive moments was so self-motivating that in time it moved from being a forced habit to a natural and free-flowing state.

The Healing Power of Gratitude
(Honoring This Given Life)

TIME NEEDED: 10 MINUTES

THIS MEDITATION WILL guide us into grateful awareness, the welcoming heart space for the beauty of our lives.

Find a comfortable place to sit and allow yourself to come into stillness.

You might close your eyes or leave them open slightly.

Now begin to notice the gentle wave of the breath as you breathe through the nose.

Let the breath soothe you as you drop into this meditation, releasing all of the worries and busyness of the day.

If there's a barrier to breathing through the nose, focus on where you can connect with the breath more naturally. Maybe you can feel its wave swell at the belly or ripple through the body.

Watch and witness as the body breathes itself.

You might begin to feel the sensations of aliveness from the inside out.

Here we will strengthen in our stillness and rewire for the kind of embodied gratitude that empowers and heals and returns us to an awakened life.

Begin to settle into the body and notice what draws the mind's attention, holding it with great wonder and a sense of natural appreciation.

The sensations in the muscles, the beating heart, the feeling of the breath, the sounds in the room, the thoughts—holding all of it in awe.

Place the hands gently at the eyes. Rest your attention there. The eyes are our gateway to the outer realms, showing us the way of the world. They trace the lines of the sunset and capture the leaf as it dances its way down to the ground. Through the eyes, we take in the smile of our dear ones and carry beauty back into our heart. The eyes show us what is painful and good in our world and return us to the sacred in all things.

Repeat these words now in a whisper, and only if they truly express what you are feeling:

I give thanks now to the gift of seeing.

Place the hands gently at the nose and remember now the perfume of the fresh sea air as it awakens you to this perfect moment. Savor now the scent of a good dense broth or the waft of sweetness that greets you as you step through the door, weary and ready to be nourished.

Repeat these words now:

I give thanks now to the gift of smell.

Place the hands gently at the mouth. Soft lips, the vibration of sound, unwinding the knots of words and delivering us from the unconscious places we have been lodged. The mouth nourishes and loves and holds a firm "no." It transmutes truth and makes our voice heard.

I give thanks now to the gift of voice.

Place the hands gently at the ears. The whispers of the wind, the cry of a newborn baby, the timbres of strings plucked, voices heard, the gift of sound arriving at the ear as if to say, "Here you are, listen now to the sacred accord. It sings for you."

I give thanks now to the gift of hearing.

Place the hands gently at the heart. The heart beats faithfully 100,000 times in the turn of a day. It saves lives, ends wars, endures grief, and returns us to that which is pure and good even when we feel most shattered. Let us gladly give over to the wisdom of the heart, leading us to one another.

I give thanks now to the gift of the heart.

Place the hands together and feel now the aliveness of your life force between the fingers. Hold with gratitude the strength and the capability of these tender hands. Feel the sensation of your essence vibrating and radiating through.

I give thanks now to the gift of these hands, holding source, eternally grateful for this given life.

May you dwell in the current of gratitude until the deliberate effort of practice drops away and its intention begins to flow into the natural joy of your own wise heart.

Breathe, notice, and be.

Shona's Story: Afterword

"Do you have a sense of why the lotus is showing itself to you now?" I'd asked Shona. She was trying to focus on the "little wins," she said. Losing her baby was the worst pain she had ever experienced and it changed her whole outlook on life. Appreciating moments of lightness and joy helped to release her from grief, a reprieve that she greatly welcomed. She was grateful for the grace of healing and the unwavering support of her friends. Gradually the beauty of the world began to show itself once again and she looked at it with a renewed sense of awe. Shona found light in the darkness. And she thought the lotus was a perfect symbol for her healing.

Top 3 Takeaways

1. When practiced over time, gratitude rewires our mind-body system for a happier, healthier life. Taking the time to sit in appreciation for the moments of contentment, joy, and respect for this given life moves us from a mind-set of lacking to one of abundance.

2. Gratitude is more than a fleeting feeling. It's a soul quality, a lived embodiment of a higher, kinder intelligence, and a powerful instigator to a more peaceful, emotionally and physically healthy life.

3. In time, gratitude is no longer a practice that requires effort to think of or do. Instead, it's a natural embodiment of loving awareness.

Journal Prompts

- Take a few minutes every evening this week to sit quietly and reflect on three things that went well and why they went well. They need not be big events; simple things will do. Record the three events in a journal or on a device. Making a record is important to this exercise. As the week comes to an end, reflect on the impact of pausing each day to sit in appreciation for the moments of contentment, joy, and respect for this given life. Do you remember the lotus story? Reflect too on the gifts that were born from those difficult times in your life— this is where we learn to appreciate the gifts in the muck.

- You can deepen your practice by using the eight soul qualities of gratitude as a framework for your gratitude journaling. You need not address them all, just choose the ones that speak to you the most on any given day.

- Awe: What did you experience, big or small, that inspired you today? It could be something you saw, heard, or otherwise experienced. Instead of focusing on what you may have accomplished or ticked off on your to-do list, bring your heart and mind to a moment of wonder for the ordinary exquisiteness of life.

- Appreciation of the present moment: What small blessing exists right in front of you, right now? What are you rejecting about this moment? What might it be like to be fully present in the moment and open to what it may be teaching?

- Internal abundance: What are you thankful for in your body or inner world? Your health? Your beating heart? Your breath? Your inner knowing? Your intuition? Explain why.

- Compassionate comparison: Write about someone you know who is experiencing difficulty right now and sink deeply into the wish that they are relieved of their hardship. Consider whether you might be able to support them in some way. If so, take a moment to appreciate that you have the strength and fortitude to do so.

- Appreciation of others: Connect now to someone in your life who's been kind to you. Let the mind rest on an ordinary event. Perhaps your partner unloaded the dishwasher so you could have a much-needed bath. Or a coworker brought you a cup of tea at your desk in the middle of the afternoon. Describe how that small act of support influenced you and the core feelings that emerged. Notice too whether the mind generates stories: that their small act of kindness was overdue or not enough or tainted by ulterior motives. Return to embracing and validating the goodness of that one small gesture.

- The wisdom of adversity: Write about something you've lost or thought you wanted and then had to release. Or you might write about a difficulty from the past or present. What did you learn about yourself? In what ways did you grow? This learning doesn't need to be a major revelation—most aren't. Look for small discoveries.

- The power of ritual: How will you make authentic and embodied gratitude a part of your daily rituals? What are some concrete ways you can achieve this?

- Oneness: Describe a time you felt a sense of wonder for this big interdependent human family. You may have had that feeling while enjoying nature or at a family celebration or perhaps during meditation. What are some simple ways you could attune to the oneness and take small steps toward supporting the greater good of the whole?

Mama Space

Self-Realization and Motherhood

"Once we release our fears as a parent we can walk with our children as their students and fellow-travelers. This is the ultimate purpose of parenting."

DR. SHEFALI

Emma's Story

"Not one person told me that when I had kids I'd be judged either for being a working mom or for staying at home with the kids. And they certainly didn't let me in on the fact that when push comes to shove, my career will always come second," Emma told me. She'd started to come for counseling several months after her children's school shut down in-person classes due to an outbreak of COVID-19. Her husband had always been supportive of her career as an event planner for a major women's clothing retail company. It was meaningful work, and the additional income took the heat off living in the most expensive city in Canada. Before the pandemic, they had just found that sweet spot of career and family balance: they had childcare in place, most nights both parents made it home for family dinner, and both kids and parents seemed to be feeling fulfilled. Then the pandemic hit and Emma left her job to stay home with the kids.

"Someone needs to literally sit right beside the girls while they do their homework. By the time my husband gets home, I'm absolutely done. I'm hearing the same story with so many of my friends. I'm the lower-income earner, so guess who gets to give up her career to cook and clean and homeschool the kids?" There was no silver lining. The most important thing I could do for Emma in that moment was to lean in and listen hard, honor her, and validate her anger for being caught along the fault lines of gender inequality. She continued, "Have you heard the term 'shecession'!?" I hadn't. "You should read about it: men are either holding on to their jobs or bouncing back into the workforce while women are leaving the workforce in droves to fall back into being the caregivers! Women are being set back decades, and I'm pissed!"

Emma's was an understandable rage, the kind of anger that could set up residence in the body. Emma had worked hard to become a parent. Years of infertility had led to rounds of intrauterine insemination, two rounds of unsuccessful in vitro fertilization, and then a successful pregnancy. She'd endured injections, hormonal fluctuations, grief and loss, and the financial pressure of fertility treatments. For Emma, becoming a mom felt like a miracle, and she'd poured herself into raising her twin girls. She loved her kids, but spending so much time together had made her feel like a bad parent. Between the social and professional isolation and the never-ending cooking, cleaning, and looking after her children, Emma was well past her threshold of coping.

"Everything feels hard right now: the planning, the coordinating, and the constant worrying. Before COVID, I was already dealing with enough. Every time the kids had a cold or a doctor's appointment, of course it was me that ended up taking time off work. I started lying to my boss and hiding the fact that I was tending to the kids. Women without children are the ones getting ahead at the company I work for. Now I'm not sure if I'll have a job to go back to." But while Emma was furious at the ways that her company's executives had ignored the conflicting demands on working parents, she didn't have the time or energy to advocate for change.

As it was for many others the pandemic was a stark reveal for Emma. It showed her where she was at in her marriage, with her children, her employer, and most of all, herself. Fears of loss of identity, self-judgment, and disempowerment were front and center—painfully so. And while she couldn't change the reality of parenting during a pandemic, she was able to mobilize her strength and honor the extraordinary role she was playing in her family's lives.

Finding Our Mama Space

I can't think of a mother who hasn't told me (in one way or another) that being a mother is an extraordinary and life-affirming experience. It can also be extremely challenging. If we are to foster an honoring and fulfilling relationship with ourselves as mothers, we need to be able to take care of ourselves and each other—to give ourselves profoundly compassionate attention. This chapter is your invitation to a dedicated practice of self-care and conscious mothering. It's based on mind-body health practices I have used for decades, both as a personal refuge and in my work with mothers. The meditation, mantras, and journaling questions are a path toward greater presence, fulfillment, and connection—they are systematically chosen to help narrow the gap between what the judging mind tells you should be so and what already perfectly is.

In the last few years I have had hundreds of deep-dive discussions with mothers about the things that matter most to them. I've witnessed a major shift in the collective female consciousness: a determination and a commitment to challenge the restrictive and harmful collective patterns that can lead to absolute overwhelm. We want less chaos and more tenderness. We yearn for a more compassionate relationship with our self, our partners, and especially our children. But the pressure to be all things to all people slowly, insidiously, depletes our endurance and strength. At times we feel devoured by the unconscious expectations coming at us at every turn. We feel the loss of our feminine nature, our vital resource for connecting with ourselves and those we love.

I'm in awe of the mamas working so hard to raise their children with grace and hope and consciousness. Each of you feels the weight of the task ahead, raising a next generation that is wise, compassionate, and resilient enough to heal that which needs to be healed. To do this well, we require the time and space to go deeply inward and heal ourselves.

Conscious Mothering

An idea that has gained resonance over the past decade is the concept of conscious parenting, especially in the work of Dr. Shefali, a colleague of mine who is the author of *The Conscious Parent* and *The Awakened Family*. The idea is that it is easy to fall into unhealthy patterns with our children, often using systems of rewards and punishments and trying to be in control of (and often overpower) their behavior. Conscious mothering involves removing ourselves from those patterns and doing the self-work needed to find alternatives, because knowing ourselves intimately unhooks us from the reactive unconscious patterns that can harm. The "conscious" part is being deliberate about being non-judgmental of our children, separating our ego from our parenting role and honoring their spirit.

Conscious parenting means that instead of punishing a child for acting out, we pause for a moment and consider what emotions and struggles might underlie that behavior. And while we still talk with the child about the impact of their reactions, the importance of boundaries, and the need to make better choices, we respectfully learn together. This philosophy is based on the idea that our children are also our teachers, and we are awakening our consciousness together. It is an illusion to think the "perfect mother" exists. But key to conscious parenting is that our role is to model and not to

A LITTLE NOTE OF ENCOURAGEMENT

Even when we have a strong inner sense of where we're headed, we can unwittingly send fuzzy messages. Becoming crystal clear about your bottom line clarifies to you (and those in your life) exactly what you are and aren't willing to do. These bright-line rules lead to predictable and consistent returns, transforming life for the better. They can also lead us out of harmful habits or into more supportive ones. As an example, if it's better sleep you want, your self-honoring boundary might be: "I don't drink caffeine after 3 p.m." or "I turn off technology one hour before bed." If it's time for journaling or meditation you're after, you might let your partner know: "I'm switching out our nightly Netflix time for thirty minutes of practice." When you have clear boundaries, you don't need to work quite so hard navigating daily decisions about whether something fits or doesn't. Go ahead and define your bright-line rules—they're not only helpful in meeting your goals; they are your birthright.

mold, to raise children according to their needs rather than what we need them to be. But to do this, we must attend to our own needs first. As Dr. Shefali writes in *The Conscious Parent*, "It's no surprise that we fail to tune into our children's essence. How can we listen to them when so many of us barely listen to ourselves? How can we feel their spirit and feel the beat of their heart if we can't do this in our own life?"[1]

Metta for Mothers
(Loving Kindness)

TIME NEEDED: 9 MINUTES

EMBODYING CONSCIOUS, COMPASSIONATE mothering, this Metta meditation will nourish your heart connection with your child. Metta meditation is one of the most widely researched meditations and it has been shown to improve self-acceptance, positive emotion, and relationships and to foster unity.

If you're not a parent, imagine instead a child you feel close with (or any child for that matter). We begin by focusing loving awareness for the well-being of a child, then for ourselves, and we close with kind wishes for us both. To extend the benefits of this meditation, you can move your field of loving awareness outward and take it as far as you wish. After you focus on a child and yourself, you can call to mind a benefactor—someone who has helped you—and share your words of kindness to them. One by one you can include your family, friends, colleagues, and acquaintances. Include strangers and the people you see every day without giving them much attention at all. This meditation can be extra powerful when used as a vehicle for forgiveness. If it seems hard to imagine directing loving kindness to someone who's hurt you or with whom you've had difficulty, keep in mind that you don't need to manufacture feelings that don't feel authentic. You can send these wishes of loving kindness with the hope that the person you are thinking of learns from any wrongdoings.

Feel your body where it makes contact with the support beneath you and allow yourself to settle within. Close your eyes, feel the breath entering and leaving the body, and with each exhale feel yourself sinking into the tenderness of this moment. Place your right hand on the heart and make the heart center the full focus of your attention. Feel the warmth emanating there, pure and bright. Allow it to grow until it fills the body and fills the room. Place your hands comfortably on your lap and dwell peacefully in this present moment. There is nowhere else to go and no better thing to do than this. Simply be in the vibration of that vast and healing love known as total oneness.

Now bring to mind a vision of your child standing or sitting before you. Picture them clearly and feel a great wave of tenderness between you. And now hold them in the heart and the mind and repeat these words to them:

May you be safe.
May you be happy.
May you be healthy.
May you be free of suffering.
May you live with ease.

Now bring your awareness to that same inner tenderness and this time begin to direct those same feelings of love to yourself. Focus on the sensations in and around the heart. Glow in the radiant energy of your loving kindness and repeat these words:

May I be safe.
May I be happy.
May I be healthy.
May I be free of suffering.
May I live with ease.

Begin to sense now the heart connection between you and your child. You might sense it as a ray of light connecting their heart center to yours. And while they have their own gifts and their own imprint on the world, so too are they a part of your journey of awakening. Picture now a great and healing golden light around you both.

May we be safe.
May we be happy.
May we be healthy.
May we be free of suffering.
May we live with ease.

Take a low and slow breath and gently open your eyes. Place your hand on the heart and set the intention to walk through your day with the awareness that your loving energy travels through your thoughts, your words, and your actions—it travels fast, far, and wide.

Breathe, notice, and be.

---

10 *Mantras for Mamas*

Mantra practice is ideal for busy moms. Closed-eye practice takes but a minute or two (first thing in the morning is often most realistic) and you can always recite mantras (out loud, as a whisper, or in your mind) as you bounce between school and soccer practice, during bath time, or any other time that suits you. Mantras can be an anchor in stressful times, and during those openings of quiet they can bring even greater peace.

Read through the following ten mantras and pick the one that stands out the most. You'll know it automatically. If none of the mantras resonate, you might create your own or draw on the mantras in chapter 6. The healing and empowering impact of mantras is built over time. Consider sticking with one for now and allow it to do its work.

My child is my sacred contract for growth

As I guide my child, they too are guiding me

My child is already whole, they need not prove their worth

I soften my eyes, my hands, my words, and my heart

My breath will guide me to a gentler, wiser way

My awakened presence is my child's greatest protection

This, too, is a perfect moment

Intentional solitude is an act of courage

My love is unconditional and infinite

The fulfillment I seek in others rests solely within me

My Motherhood Story

As is the case for many women, becoming a mother wasn't easy for me. I returned from my honeymoon pregnant, a surprise that took me from disbelief to acceptance, joy, and then despair when I miscarried. My husband and I hadn't planned to start a family so early in our marriage, but at the time I felt the grief from losing my baby could be quelled only by becoming pregnant once again. Over the next few years we found ourselves on a path of conception and loss. Each monthly period sent me reeling into feelings of inadequacy, convinced my body was betraying me. After my having spent so many years trying to prevent pregnancy, the idea that conceiving could be so hard seemed unimaginable. Other women seemed to float through pregnancy without any difficulties, and I imagined they were all sharing in a sacred experience I would never have. While a wiser part of me knew better, I had fully bought into our society's message that if I couldn't have a child, I was broken. In my mind, they were whole and I was not.

At first I spoke very little about the miscarriages because I was too embarrassed. I felt very much alone in the pain and the sadness and the grief. But in time I found the courage to voice these emotions, and soon other women—friends and family who had never previously talked to me about infertility or miscarriage—began to share their stories of loss and soothe me with their honesty. I thought about the many women who had struggled before me. Imagine how many women in over 4 billion years of human existence have been brought to their knees through infertility or miscarriage.

After five miscarriages, I became pregnant again. Instead of celebrating, I became hypervigilant about every twinge, cramp, and Braxton-Hicks contraction that moved through my body. My doctor had warned me that I was at risk for delivering prematurely, and so only very late in my pregnancy did I begin to breathe more freely. The birth of my first son was a joy unlike anything else I had known. And each day after that was filled with the kind of natural gratitude that grows only when one knows hardship intimately. The pain of our previous losses dissolved in his smiles, and grief dominated my thoughts less and less.

When we decided to try and grow our family, I was less fretful about the negative pregnancy tests and even the miscarriages seemed more manageable. After all, I had a preschooler to distract me. Then, after the birth of my second son, something shifted and I found myself in a darkness I'd never known before. I obsessed about my children's schedules, lay awake at night going through lists of tasks for the next day, and felt a sense of dread so heavy I could barely breathe. No amount of meditation, breath work, or therapy could lift the panic that I woke up to and lived with throughout the day. What I didn't understand at the time is that I was suffering from a form of postpartum depression rarely identified until recently: postpartum anxiety.

Postpartum depression is typically characterized by feelings of sadness, irritability, tearfulness, changes in appetite, and disturbed sleep, but those weren't my symptoms at all. And while new mothers recognize they're feeling out of balance, they assume the lack of sleep, racing thoughts, and need for control are just regular stressors that all new mothers face. That belief—and the message many of us have internalized that we need to be superwomen solving every problem ourselves—prevents many of us from asking for help. But we must learn to do so. We simply can't look after other people effectively unless we also look after ourselves.

Here are some facts every new mother should know about post-partum imbalance from the Anxiety and Depression Association of America.

- 13% of new mothers experience postpartum depression
- 3–5% experience postpartum obsessive-compulsive disorder
- 9% experience postpartum post-traumatic stress disorder associated with pregnancy or childbirth
- 6% of pregnant women and 10% of postpartum women experience clinical levels of anxiety[2]

While these serious conditions usually develop between one and three weeks after delivery, they often aren't identified until much later. So look for warning signs early, and don't hesitate to reach out to your professional support systems if you're unsure about whether you're experiencing typical emotional and physical adjustments or have crossed the threshold into postpartum anxiety (or depression).
Here's what to look for:

- constant worry
- a feeling of dread or that something bad might happen
- obsessive and irrational thinking patterns
- loss of appetite or voracious appetite
- extreme restlessness
- dizziness, racing heart, nausea, or lack of connection with the body
- sleep disturbance (I know—what new mom doesn't face sleep disruption!?)

Regardless of whether you have a family history of postpartum or other mental health struggles, it can be deeply honoring to ask a friend or family member to help you with a postdelivery care plan.

(You can also enlist your partner for this role, but they may need a care plan themselves.) Write down what you most need and who can be of help.

In most developing cultures, postpartum disorders are virtually nonexistent largely because of the conscious and protective social structures put in place for new moms.[3] Classic anthropological research shows these structures include recognizing a distinct postpartum period, rituals of caring for the new mother, mandated rest and a reprieve from social expectations, support with the day-to-day family operations, and recognition of the sacred role of the mother (aka mothering the mother).[4] Ours, however, is a strange culture that fails to provide support and care for new moms.[5] Women continue to be the primary caregivers in families, and new mothers rarely have anyone to help at home. Our partners are usually back to work within a few weeks, and we're left to figure everything out on our own without the support systems our ancestors cultivated.

What if we had a circle of people who took turns placing soup on our stovetop until we were strengthened once again? What if we did the same in their time of need? What if we supported new moms with the practices you've discovered through the pages of this book to nourish and nurture them during this sacred and life-changing time? What if we came together with great compassion and supported new moms with our collective strength and wisdom?

Emma's Story: Afterword

Through simple practices like mantra, forgiveness meditations, and a whole lot of time in nature, Emma discovered some pathways toward greater peace in uncertain times. She leaned hard into practices to soothe her nervous system and externalized hot emotions like fear and anger by writing them out in a journal and doing breath work religiously. In time she was able to find that spaciousness where pain and pleasure can exist together—a sense of acceptance that happens when you're willing to let go, knowing that you just can't struggle against what's happening any longer. She also scheduled peace talks with her husband where they navigated parenting responsibilities together, breaking down and transcending the gender roles they had fallen into. Emma began sharing her experiences and led the way for other women to do the same. The difficulty of balancing career and family opened a gateway for Emma to learn how to meet her edge, steady herself, and greet the unknowns with a lighter heart.

Top 3 Takeaways

1. Motherhood is a deeply tender time in which we are catapulted into self-growth. The paradox is that new mothers need just as much love and care as they're giving to their new baby.

2. Motherhood is a chance to learn the true sense of what it means to be perfectly imperfect. Be kind. It's perfectly OK to feel tired, have oatmeal in our hair and for our children to be wearing mismatched socks.

3. Our children are whole and deeply wise: they are our greatest teachers, awakening us to our true selves.

Journal Prompts

- Bring to mind the strongest childhood memories you have of your mother. What do you remember about her struggles? What do you remember about her strengths?

- What unconscious patterns from the past might be repeating in your relationship with your child?

- What did you dream for yourself when you first entered motherhood? What did you dream for your child? How have these dreams crystallized into expectations?

- How can you actively embrace the difficult moments and play more, laugh more, and cultivate an ecosystem of joy for yourself and your child?

14

Rise

Stillness

When we are still enough, long enough
we begin to see what is there.
Sadness, joy, shame, fear
all waiting in the chambers of the heart
longing to be seen, heard, held.

You could not have known what was building behind the fog
of the doing, striving, proving.
You could not see until the stillness awakened you
like the sun awakens the bud to flower.

But you cannot force the bloom.

May you rest in your stillness.
May you soften your effort.
And may you discover yourself again.
Radiant, pure, light.

MICHELE KAMBOLIS

OUR LIVES ARE an unending plain of vast unknowns, a training ground for letting go and coming home: letting go of who we thought we were (or were told we should be) and coming home to the beautiful truth of who we have been all along. As we continue, we will still have times when we're less than mindful, fall out of awareness, and lose sight of our deepest intentions. So, too, will we find ourselves slipping back into old reactive patterns, knowingly neglecting the practices we know serve us best. But the most significant moments in this journey of self-realization come when we look at everything in our lives as an invitation to awaken.

Awakening to life and ourselves doesn't mean we suddenly feel free from stress and heartbreak; instead, our armor is pierced and the heart feels pain and joy with a new intensity. And when we find we've met our edge we stay there, knowing that this is our prime time for educating the heart. We understand that in our darkest of times we can look up at the gray sky and know that on the other side of those clouds lies the sun. And so we'll wait out those times with greater patience recognizing well the impermanence of every storm.

When we live in the flow of life supported by the balancing forces of nature, the tasks and relationships and decisions we face daily become less daunting. An intuitive wisdom moves through us and lifts us up to navigate the groundlessness. Fear dissolves, life happens, and we soar along. We discover the natural rhythm of this beautiful and chaotic life. We look after ourselves and practice self-compassion, sleep well, and eat in ways that show respect to our body. As we find our natural balance through meditation, writing, creating, sustenance, ritual, connection, nature, and other nourishing practices, we find ourselves more self-accepting, openhearted, and available in ways that seemed impossible before. We develop a natural desire to clear the clouds of suffering with organized and inspired action that cultivates real and lasting change. And we find ourselves with the energy that is needed to heal and harmonize the world around us.

As you heal, awaken, and transform, the shifts in your emotional, mental, and physical reality spread throughout humanity. As one person heals, we all begin to heal. It's like the catchphrase from that Fabergé Organics shampoo commercial of the early '80s in which the model with shimmering, healthy hair told two friends about it and they told two friends, and so on, and so on, and so on.

When we have the strength and resilience to meet life where it's at, we find ourselves opening to even the most difficult of situations with the courage to stay there. Inwardly, we stop running, hiding, and changing ourselves to become what we've been told we should be. We understand that we never needed to be fixed in the first place and that our life is not a self-improvement project but a path of rediscovery. Each new day is an invitation to abandon self-criticism and shed our cultural baggage so we can live with unwavering self-compassion, know the spirit of inner goodness, and begin to soar beyond the boundaries of the conditioned mind to feel the expansiveness of life itself. And we want deeply the same for others.

Instead of judging and complaining and creating a story in difficult times, we learn to soften into a situation with greater understanding and compassion. When someone barks at us, criticizes, or ignores us altogether, we might pause a little more often and take it less personally. We might think back to times when we too were angry or anxious or harmful, and look at the current situation with a little more patience and understanding. From this place of interconnectedness, we see there is no "I" or "you" or "them." We are a single transcendent force—described by saints and mystics since the beginning of time—and we sense it whenever we create or meditate or connect into love.

Maya Angelou once said, "There is no greater agony than bearing an untold story inside of you." Throughout this book, you've had the opportunity to look at your life intimately and you've learned some new ways to practice wise and gentle living and steadily strengthen your innate healing capacities. I hope you have grown into your self-knowing, are pausing a little more often, and feel yourself living out your wisdom and inner truth. It can take an enormous amount of courage to overcome our fear of truly being known. If you have a message burning from within, this is your invitation to become bold and fearless, a heart warrior for these times. We've held on tight to the safety of silence, but the winds have come and opened our lungs to speak of a wiser way.

So take a moment now to turn inward and begin to ask:

How will I use my voice to help shape these times?

What impact might I have if I revealed more, said more, shared more?

What gifts am I ready to actualize?

What intention can I set right now to mobilize the message moving through me?

A LITTLE NOTE OF ENCOURAGEMENT

I'm deeply honored that you chose to embark on this courageous journey with me, and may the science and soul of this book support you in the unending process of awakening. May you use the practices each day, no matter what's happening in your life. Over time they will inspire a level of fulfillment beyond what you've been told is possible. As you continue to awaken and rise, may you carry a freedom of spirit that meets the heartbreak and uncertainties of life with compassion and courage wholeheartedly.

As you rise, we all rise.

Love and Radiance Meditation

TIME NEEDED: 10 MINUTES

THIS MEDITATION WILL open the gateway to your innermost being with great clarity. You'll activate a powerful healing wisdom that will return you to the truth that you have always been enough. Fear, self-judgment, and anxiety can no longer thrive in this place of free-flowing love. And in the spirit of our greatest goodness, may we wish the same for all others.

Remember, meditation is available to you anywhere, any time. It asks only that you be willing.

Let's begin.

Turn inward by closing your eyes and remember there is no better use of time today than this, a time to pause in quiet stillness, a time to come home to the essence of you—the beautiful light that you were born as: infinite love and pure goodness.

Breathe naturally through the nose, accepting each breath as it is. If it's shallow, let it be shallow; if it's deep, let it be deep. Since the moment of your first breath the body has known what to do.

Breathe and illuminate as love.

With each new breath, notice the miracle of the body breathing. Each inhale brings you into the beauty of this new moment: present time. This moment is your highest place of power, where the past is no more and the future has not yet arrived. Rest. For in life as it is here, you may lay down the compulsion to strive and prove and acquire your worth. The rose need not explain its beauty; it simply receives the rain and wind and light as they meet its soft petals.

Breathe and illuminate as love.

Bring your attention to the sensations at the heart center and choose to soften into this beautiful gift of life you've been given. It's time to move beyond the harshness of what you've been told, the interwoven messages that you're somehow not enough. How can a soul be anything less than sacred when it is created from source and nature itself? I know the hurt you carry comparing yourself with others as if one soaring eagle were somehow better than another.

Breathe and illuminate as love.

May I remind you to rebel against the idea of external beauty as a standard for your worth. May you drop the heavy stones you've been told to carry, each one weighted with the message that you must somehow earn your worth. We must learn to live more wisely and choose only that which leads us back to love.

Breathe and illuminate as love.

With each breath and each heartbeat may you dissolve all of the parables and myths you've inherited from those who were lost themselves. Within you still lies a wide-eyed child trying to confirm that she is worthy of being seen. May you cloak her in the healing fabric of compassion and may your eyes affirm, "You are grace, you are light, you are goodness. Be as you are."

Breathe and illuminate as love.

On the twenty-third day after your conception your heart began to beat, and day by day it became stronger. In each moment of your life it has sustained you faithfully. It asks nothing. Offer your heart center the full focus of your attention now, placing the hands against the heart and feeling deeply the power source that makes this life possible. From the heart flows a current of limitless love and compassion, pure and bright.

Breathe and illuminate as love.

Through each breath, each moment of loving awareness, you have everything you need. Right here, right now. You are whole. With each inhale, breathe in these words holding them as your own:

I am thankful for this breath,
this body, and this life.
I am grateful for who I am
and how far I've come.
All that I need
resides in this moment alone.
And in each breath
I lead myself back to brilliant self-love.

Inhale with the awareness that self-love is grace, it is joy, and it is your own brilliant power.

It is your healing. It is your strength. It is the core essence of you. It is yours.

Breathe and illuminate as love.

Concluding Intention

May we open to trust that this life is beating for us.

May we steady ourselves with a wisdom built on 4 billion years of life lived.

May we gaze inward and avail ourselves of the teachings of this time.

May we be fueled by a wellspring of compassion and courage.

Let us never forget the vastness of our own spirit and may we rise together.

Acknowledgments

MANY PEOPLE HELPED me bring this book to life. Their commitment and dedication to this project have moved me beyond measure.

My profound appreciation goes to Chris Labonté for believing wholeheartedly in this book. And to Lara Smith for keeping me on track and providing steady support.

I would also like to send my sincere thanks to Lesley Cameron, who has been a brilliant and very patient editor. We edited version after version until the words flowed in ways that danced right into our hearts.

My sincere thanks to Lucy Kenward for her keen eye, Alex Kambolis for collating hundreds of research articles, and Naomi MacDougall for a design that captures the essence of the book so beautifully.

Thank you to Sarah Bancroft, who played an essential role in the evolution of this book. And Jim Tobler, who also made invaluable contributions.

Many thanks to Alyssa Bauman, a wonderful friend and expert nutritionist, for providing her support and guidance for the chapter on sustenance.

My heartfelt gratitude to my mom for her unwavering love. And to my family (Alex, Stamos, Jamie, and Lloyd) for bringing a joy to my life that soars beyond words.

Finally, I wish to extend sincere appreciation for the teachings of Tara Brach, Pema Chödrön, Jack Kornfield, Sharon Salzberg, Dr. Shefali, and the many other wisdom teachers who've inspired and guided me along the dharmic path. And to Ram Dass, who opened my heart in ways I hadn't known possible.

Notes

CHAPTER 1: STRESS: PHYSICAL, MENTAL, SPIRITUAL

1   Rachel Yehuda and Amy Lehrner, "Intergenerational Transmission of Trauma Effects:
    Putative Role of Epigenetic Mechanisms," *World Psychiatry* 17, no. 3 (October 2018):
    243–57, doi:10.1002/wps.20568.

2   H. B. Simpson et al., *Anxiety Disorders: Theory, Research, and Clinical Perspectives*
    (New York City: Columbia University, 2010).

3   "Any Anxiety Disorder," Mental Health Information: Statistics, National Institute of
    Mental Health, November 2017, www.nimh.nih.gov/health/statistics/any-anxiety
    -disorder.shtml.

4   Carmen P. McLean et al., "Gender Differences in Anxiety Disorders: Prevalence,
    Course of Illness, Comorbidity and Burden of Illness," *Journal of Psychiatric
    Research* 45, no. 8 (August 2011): 1027–35, doi:10.1016/j.jpsychires.2011.03.006.

5   A. P. Borrow and R. J. Handa, "Estrogen Receptors Modulation of Anxiety-Like
    Behavior," *Vitamins and Hormones* 103 (October 2016): 27–52, doi:10.1016/
    bs.vh.2016.08.004.

6   "Violence against Women: A 'Global Health Problem of Epidemic Proportions,'" WHO
    Media Centre, World Health Organization, June 20, 2013, www.who.int/mediacentre/
    news/releases/2013/violence_against_women_20130620/en/.

7   "Violence against Women."

8   "Child Marriage: Late Trends and Future Prospects," UNICEF Resources, United
    Nations International Children's Emergency Fund, July 2018, data.unicef.org/
    resources/child-marriage-latest-trends-and-future-prospects/.

9   "The World's Women 2015: Trends and Statistics," UN Department of Economic
    and Social Affairs, United Nations, 2015, unstats.un.org/unsd/gender/downloads/
    worldswomen2015_report.pdf.

10 "Global Wage Growth Lowest Since 2008, While Women Still Earning 20 Per Cent Less
    than Men," ILO Newsroom, International Labour Organization, November 26, 2018,
    www.ilo.org/moscow/news/WCMS_650551/lang--en/index.htm.

11 "Women in Politics: 2019," IPU Knowledge, Inter-Parliamentary Union, 2019,
    www.ipu.org/resources/publications/infographics/2019-03/women-in-politics-2019.

12 "Fast Facts: Statistics on Violence against Women and Girls," UN Women:
    Programming Essentials, Monitoring & Evaluation, UN Women, October 31, 2010,
    www.endvawnow.org/en/articles/299-fast-facts-statistics-on-violence-against
    -women-and-girls.html.

13 "Women, Business and the Law 2019: A Decade of Reform," International Bank for
    Reconstruction and Development, The World Bank Group, 2019, openknowledge
    .worldbank.org/bitstream/handle/10986/31327/WBL2019.pdf.

14 Angela Y. Davis, *Women, Race & Class* (New York City: Random House, Inc., 1981).

15 Rich Simon, "An Interview with Peter Levine," *Psychotherapy Networker*
    (March/April 2019), www.psychotherapynetworker.org/magazine/article/2347/
    an-interview-with-peter-levine.

16 Evert Boonstra et al., "Neurotransmitters as Food Supplements: The Effects of GABA
    on Brain and Behavior," *Frontiers in Psychology* 6 (October 2015): 1520, doi:0.3389/
    fpsyg.2015.01520.

17 Megan Galbally et al., "The Role of Oxytocin in Mother-Infant Relations: A Systematic
    Review of Human Studies," *Harvard Review of Psychology* 19, no. 1 (January/
    February 2011): 1–14, doi:10.3109/10673229.2011.549771.

18 "Blood Sugar & Stress," Types of Diabetes, University of California, San Francisco,
    2021, dtc.ucsf.edu/types-of-diabetes/type2/understanding-type-2-diabetes/
    how-the-body-processes-sugar/blood-sugar-stress/.

19 Hilda Wong et al., "The Effects of Mental Stress on Non-Insulin-Dependent Diabetes: Determining the Relationship between Catecholamine and Adrenergic Signals from Stress, Anxiety, and Depression on the Physiological Changes in the Pancreatic Hormone Secretion," *Cureus* 11, no. 8 (August 2019): e5474, doi:10.7759/cureus.5474.

20 Firdaus S. Dhabhar, "The Short-Term Stress Response—Mother Nature's Mechanism for Enhancing Protection and Performance under Conditions of Threat, Challenge, and Opportunity," *Frontiers in Neuroendocrinology* 49 (April 2018): 175–92, doi:10.1016/j.yfrne.2018.03.004.

21 "Chronic Stress Puts Your Health at Risk," Mayo Clinic, March 19, 2019, www.mayoclinic.org/healthy-lifestyle/stress-management/in-depth/stress/art-20046037.

22 "Any Anxiety Disorder."

CHAPTER 2: HEALING: OUR INNATE ABILITY TO HEAL

1   "Unlock the Power of Your Heart," HeartMath, www.heartmath.com.

2   Friedhelm Stetter and Sirko Kuppter, "Autogenic Training: A Meta-Analysis of Clinical Outcome Studies," *Applied Psychophysiology and Biofeedback* 27, no. 1 (March 2002): 45–98, doi:10.1023/a:1014576505223.

3   Gian Mauro Manzoni et al., "Relaxation Training for Anxiety: A Ten-Years Systematic Review with Meta-Analysis," *BMC Psychiatry* 8, no. 41 (June 2008), doi:10.1186/1471-244X-8-41.

4   E. Jacobson, "You Must Relax," *Medicine* (1963), doi:10.2307/1415769.

5   P. M. Scheufele, "Effects of Progressive Relaxation and Classical Music on Measurements of Attention, Relaxation, and Stress Responses," *Journal of Behavioral Medicine* 23, no. 2 (April 2000): 207–28, doi:10.1023/a:1005542121935.

6   Kai Liu et al., "Effects of Progressive Muscle Relaxation on Anxiety and Sleep Quality in Patients with COVID-19," *Complementary Therapies in Clinical Practice* 39 (May 2020), doi:10.1016/j.ctcp.2020.101132.

7   Peir Hossein Koulivand, Maryam Khaleghi Ghadiri, and Ali Gorji, "Lavender and the Nervous System," *Evidence Based-Complementary and Alternative Medicine* 2013 (March 2013), doi:10.1155/2013/681304.

CHAPTER 3: MEDITATION: A GATEWAY TO WELL-BEING

1   Daniel Goleman and Richard Davidson, *Altered Traits: Science Reveals How Meditation Changes Your Mind, Brain, and Body* (New York City: Avery Publishing, 2017), 336.

2   Madhav Goyal et al., "Meditation Programs for Psychological Stress and Well-Being: A Systematic Review and Meta-Analysis," *Journal of the American Medical Association* 174, no. 3 (March 2014): 357–68, doi:10.1001/jamainternmed.2013.13018.

3   Britta K. Holzel et al., "Differential Engagement of Anterior Cingulate and Adjacent Medial Frontal Cortex in Adept Meditators and Non-Meditators," *Neuroscience Letters* 421, no. 1 (June 2007): 16–21, doi:10.1016/j.neulet.2007.04.074.

4   Eileen Luders et al., "The Unique Brain Anatomy of Meditation Practitioners: Alterations in Cortical Gyrification," *Frontiers in Human Neuroscience* 6 (February 2012): 34, doi: 10.3389/fnhum.2012.00034.

5   Kristin D. Neff and Emma Seppälä, "Compassion, Well-Being, and the Hypoegoic Self," *Self-Compassion*, 2021, self-compassion.org/wp-content/uploads/2017/01/Neff-Seppala-chap-compassion-in-press.pdf.

6   F. Zeidan et al., "Mindfulness Meditation-Related Pain Review: Evidence for Unique Brain Mechanisms in the Regulation of Pain," *Neuroscience Letters* 520, no. 2 (June 2012): 165–73, doi:10.1016/j.neulet.2012.03.082.

7   Daniel Goleman and Richard Davidson, *Altered Traits*, 336.

8   Lidia Zylowska et al., "Mindfulness Meditation Training in Adults and Adolescents with ADHD: A Feasibility Study," *Journal of Attention Disorders* 11, no. 6 (2008): 737–46, doi:10.1177/1087054707308502.

9   Robert H. Schneider et al., "A Randomized Controlled Trial of Stress Reduction in African Americans Treated for Hypertension for over One Year," *American Journal of Hypertension* 18, no. 1 (January 2005): 88–98, doi: 10.1016/j.amjhyper.2004.08.027.

10 Laurent Valosek et al., "Effect of Meditation on Emotional Intelligence and Perceived Stress in the Workplace: A Randomized Controlled Study," *The Permanente Journal* 22 (October 2018): 17–172, doi: 10.7812/tpp/17-172.

11 Tad T. Brunyé et al., "Learning to Relax: Evaluating Four Brief Interventions for Overcoming the Negative Emotions Accompanying Math Anxiety," *Learning and Individual Differences* 27 (October 2013): 1–7, doi: 10.1016/j.lindif.2013.06.008.

12 Claire M. Zedelius and Jonathan W. Schooler, "Mind Wandering 'Ahas' Versus Mindful Reasoning: Alternative Routes to Creative Solutions," *Frontiers in Psychology* 6 (June 2015), doi: 10.3389/fpsyg.2015.00834.

13 Danah Henriksen et al., "Mindfulness and Creativity: Implications for Thinking and Learning," *Thinking Skills and Creativity* 37 (September 2020), doi:10.1016/j.tsc.2020.100689.

14 R. Gina Silverstein et al., "Effects of Mindfulness Training on Body Awareness to Sexual Stimuli: Implications for Female Sexual Dysfunction," *Psychosomatic Medicine* 73, no. 9 (November 2011): 817–25, doi:10.1097/PSY.0b013e318234e628.

15 Eileen Luders et al., "The Underlying Anatomical Correlates of Long-Term Meditation: Larger Hippocampal and Frontal Volumes of Gray Matter," *Neuroimage* 45, no. 3 (April 2009): 672–78, doi: 10.1016/j.neuroimage.2008.12.061.

CHAPTER 4: PRESENCE: MINDFULNESS AND EQUANIMITY

1   Andrea Smorti and Chiara Fioretti, "Why Narrating Changes Memory: A Contribution to an Integrative Model of Memory and Narrative Processes," *Integrative Psychological and Behavioural Science* 50 (October 2015): 296–319, doi:10.1007/s12124-015-9330-6.

2   Matthew A. Killingsworth and Daniel T. Gilbert, "A Wandering Mind Is an Unhappy Mind," *Science* 330, no. 6006 (November 2010): 932, doi:10.1126/science.1192439.

3   Jean M. Twenge, Liqing Zhang, and Charles Im, "It's Beyond My Control: A Cross-Temporal Meta-Analysis of Increasing Externality in Locus of Control, 1960–2002," *Personality and Social Psychology Review* 8, no. 3 (2004): 308–19, doi:10.1207/s15327957pspr0803_5.

4   Jean M. Twenge, Liqing Zhang, and Charles Im, "It's Beyond My Control."

5   Chet C. Sherwood, Francys Subiaul, and Tadeusz W. Zawidzki, "A Natural History of the Human Mind: Tracing Evolutionary Changes in Brain and Cognition," *Journal of Anatomy* 212, no. 4 (April 2008): 426–54, doi:10.1111/j.1469-7580.2008.00868.x.

6   Erik Wallmark et al., "Promoting Altruism through Meditation: An 8-Week Randomized Controlled Pilot Study," *Mindfulness* 4 (June 2012): 223–34, doi:10.1007/s12671-012-0115-4.

7   Daniel Goleman and Richard Davidson, *Altered Traits: Science Reveals How Meditation Changes Your Mind, Brain, and Body* (New York City: Avery Publishing, 2017), 336.

8   Offir Laufer, David Israeli, and Rony Paz, "Behavioral and Neural Mechanisms of Overgeneralization in Anxiety," *Current Biology* 26, no. 6 (March 2016): 713–22, doi:10.1016/j.cub.2016.01.023.

9   Helen Y. Weng et al., "Compassion Training Alters Altruism and Neural Response to Suffering," *Psychological Science* 24, no. 7 (July 2013): 1171–80, doi:10.1177/0956797612469537.

10 Helen Y. Weng et al., "Compassion Training Alters Altruism and Neural Response to Suffering."

11 Elena Antonova, Paul Chadwick, and Veena Kumari, "More Meditation, Less Habituation? The Effect of Mindfulness Practice on the Acoustic Startle Reflex," *PLOS ONE* 10, no. 5 (May 2015), doi:10.1371/journal.pone.0123512.

12 Judson A. Brewer et al., "Meditation Experience Is Associated with Differences in Default Mode Network Activity and Connectivity," *Proceedings of the National Academy of Sciences of the United States of America* 108, no. 50 (December 2011): 20254–59, doi:10.1073/pnas.1112029108.

13 Alan S. Cowen and Dacher Keltner, "Self-Report Captures 27 Distinct Categories of Emotion Bridged by Continuous Gradients," *Proceedings of the National Academy of Sciences of the United States of America* 114, no. 36 (September 2017), doi:10.1073/pnas.1702247114.

CHAPTER 5: BREATH: OUR SUPERPOWER

1   Andrea Zaccaro et al., "How Breath-Control Can Change Your Life: A Systematic Review on Psycho-Physiological Correlates of Slow Breathing," *Frontiers in Human Neuroscience* 12 (September 2018): 353, doi:10.3389/fnhum.2018.00353.

2   Xiao Ma et al., "The Effect of Diaphragmatic Breathing on Attention, Negative Affect and Stress in Healthy Adults," *Frontiers in Psychology* 8 (June 2017): 874, doi:10.3389/fpsyg.2017.00874.

3   George M. Dallam and Bethany Kies, "The Effect of Nasal Breathing Versus Oral and Oronasal Breathing during Exercise: A Review," *Journal of Sports Research* 7, no. 1 (January 2020): 1–10, doi:10.18488/journal.90.2020.71.1.10.

4   Syed S. Mahmood et al., "The Framingham Heart Study and the Epidemiology of Cardiovascular Diseases: A Historical Perspective," *The Lancet* 383, no. 9921 (March 2014): 999–1008, doi:10.1016/S0140-6736(13)61752-3.

5   "New Survey Takes a Peek into Americans' Bedrooms to Reveal What's Keeping People Awake: Mouth Breathing," GlaxoSmithKline Consumer Healthcare, Cision PR Newswire, March 4, 2015, www.prnewswire.com/news-releases/new-survey-takes-a-peek-into-americans-bedrooms-to-reveal-whats-keeping-people-awake-mouth-breathing-300044836.html.

6   "Research on Sudarshan Kriya," The Art of Living blog, 2021, www.artofliving.org/us-en/research-sudarshan-kriya-old.

CHAPTER 6: SONG AND MANTRA: THE HEALING POTENTIAL OF SOUND

1   Hari Sharma, "Meditation: Process and Effects," *Ayu* 36, no. 3 (July 2015): 233–37, doi: 10.4103/0974-8520.182756.

2   René Pierre Le Scouarnec et al., "Use of Binaural Beat Tapes for Treatment of Anxiety: A Pilot Study of Tape Preference and Outcomes," *Alternative Therapies in Health and Medicine* 7, no. 1 (February 2001): 58–63.

3   Tamara L. Goldsby et al., "Effects of Singing Bowl Sound Meditation on Mood, Tension, and Well-Being: An Observational Study," *Journal of Evidence Based Complementary Medicine* 22, no. 3 (2017): 401–6, doi: 10.1177/2156587216668109.

CHAPTER 7: SLEEP: PRIORITIZING OUR RELATIONSHIP WITH SLEEP

1   "What Is a 'Trauma Therapist'?" FAQ, Sarah Pole LCSW, traumatherapistspain.com/faq/.

2 Michael J. Aminoff, François Boller, and Dick F. Swaab, "We Spend about One-Third of Our Life Either Sleeping or Attempting to Do So," *Handbook of Clinical Neurology* 98, (2011): vii, doi: 0.1016/B978-0-444-52006-7.00047-2.

3 Chun Seng Phua, Lata Jayaram, and Tissa Wijeratne, "Relationship between Sleep Duration and Risk Factors for Stroke," *Frontiers in Neurology* 8 (2017): 392, doi: 10.3389/fneur.2017.00392.

4 Cara A. Palmer and Candice A. Alfano, "Anxiety Modifies the Emotional Effects of Sleep Loss," *Current Opinion in Psychology* 34 (2020): 100–104, doi: 10.1016/j .copsyc.2019.12.001.

5 A. M. Williamson and Anne-Marie Feyer, "Moderate Sleep Deprivation Produces Impairments in Cognitive and Motor Performance Equivalent to Legally Prescribed Levels of Alcohol Intoxication," *Occupational and Environmental Medicine* 57, no. 10 (June 2000): 649–55.

6 Matthew Walker, *Why We Sleep: Unlocking the Power of Sleep and Dreams* (New York City: Scribner, 2017).

7 "Bedroom Poll: Summary of Findings," WB&A Market Research, National Sleep Foundation, www.sleepfoundation.org/wp-content/uploads/2018/10/NSF_Bedroom_ Poll_Report_1.pdf?x23292&x19029.

8 Rochelle Ackerley, Gaby Badre, and Hakan Olausson, "Positive Effects of a Weighted Blanket on Insomnia," *Journal of Sleep Medicine & Disorders* 2, no. 3 (2015): 1022.

9 Peir Hossein Koulivand, Maryam Khaleghi Ghadiri, and Ali Gorji, "Lavender and the Nervous System," *Evidence Based-Complementary and Alternative Medicine* 2013 (March 2013), doi:10.1155/2013/681304.

10 Namni Goel, Hyungsoo Kim, and Raymund P. Lao, "An Olfactory Stimulus Modifies Nighttime Sleep in Young Men and Women," *Chronobiology International* 22, no. 5 (2005): 889–904, doi: 0.1080/07420520500263276.

11 "Summary of Findings," WB&A Market Research, National Sleep Foundation, 2018, www.sleepfoundation.org/wp-content/uploads/2018/10/Summary_Of_Findings -FINAL.pdf.

12 Shira Polan, "Time for a Brake," *Psychology Today* (September 5, 2016), www.psychologytoday.com/ca/articles/201609/time-brake.

13 Grigorios Oikonomou et al., "The Serotonergic Raphe Promote Sleep in Zebrafish and Mice," *Neuron* 103, no. 4 (August 2019): 686–701, doi:10.1016/j.neuron.2019.05.038.

14 Vadim S. Rotenberg, "Lucid Dreams: Their Advantage and Disadvantage in the Frame of Search Activity Concept," *Frontiers in Psychology* 6 (September 2015): 1472, doi:10.3389/fpsyg.2015.01472.

15 Poppy Z. Brite, docbrite.livejournal.com/731842.html.

16 Julie Corliss, "Mindfulness Meditation Helps Fight Insomnia, Improves Sleep," Harvard Health Blog, Harvard Health Publishing, June 15, 2020, www.health .harvard.edu/blog/mindfulness-meditation-helps-fight-insomnia-improves sleep-201502187726. See also David S. Black et al., "Mindfulness Meditation and Improvement in Sleep Quality and Daytime Impairment among Older Adults with Sleep Disturbances: A Randomized Clinical Trial," *Journal of the American Medical Association* 175, no. 4 (April 2015): 494–501, doi:10.1001/jamainternmed.2014.8081.

CHAPTER 8: SUSTENANCE: FEEDING OUR WELL-BEING

1 "How Much Sugar Is Too Much?" American Heart Association, 2021, www.heart.org/ en/healthy-living/healthy-eating/eat-smart/sugar/how-much-sugar-is-too-much.

2 Dr. Siri Carpenter, "That Gut Feeling," *Monitor on Psychology* 43, no. 8 (2012): 50.

3 Dr. Siri Carpenter, "That Gut Feeling."

4   N. Litwin et al., "Consumption of Fermented Plant Foods Is Associated with Systematic Differences in the Human Gut Microbiome and Metabolome," *Current Developments in Nutrition* 4 (2020): 1573, doi:10.1093/cdn/nzaa062_030.

5   Dorin Harpaz et al., "Measuring Artificial Sweeteners Toxicity Using a Bioluminescent Bacterial Panel," *Molecules* 23, no. 10 (September 2018): 2454, doi: 10.3390/molecules23102454.

6   Mayo Clinic Staff, "Caffeine: How Much Is Too Much?," Mayo Clinic, 2021, www.mayoclinic.org/healthy-lifestyle/nutrition-and-healthy-eating/in-depth/caffeine/art-20045678.

7   Daniele Wikoff et al., "Systematic Review of the Potential Adverse Effects of Caffeine Consumption in Healthy Adults, Pregnant Women, Adolescents, and Children," *Food and Chemical Toxicology* 109, no. 1 (November 2017): 585–648, doi: 10.1016/j.fct.2017.04.002.

8   Andrew M. Taylor and Hannah D. Holscher, "A Review of Dietary and Microbial Connections to Depression, Anxiety, and Stress," *Nutritional Neuroscience* 23, no. 3 (March 2020): 237–50, doi: 10.1080/1028415X.2018.1493808.

9   Felice N. Jacka et al., "Association of Western and Traditional Diets with Depression and Anxiety in Women," *American Journal of Psychiatry* 167, no. 3 (March 2010): 305–11, doi:10.1176/appi.ajp.2009.09060881.

10 Health Canada, "Magnesium," September 1978, Updated November 1987, www.canada.ca/en/health-canada/services/publications/healthy-living/guidelines-canadian-drinking-water-quality-supporting-documents-magnesium.html.

11 Janice K. Kiecolt-Glaser et al., "Omega-3 Supplementation Lowers Inflammation and Anxiety in Medical Students: A Randomized Controlled Trial," *Brain, Behavior, and Immunity* 25, no. 8 (July 2011): 1725–34, doi: 10.1016/j.bbi.2011.07.229.

12 Kuan-Pin Su et al., "Association of Omega-3 Polyunsaturated Fatty Acids with Anxiety Symptom Severity," *Journal of the American Medicine Association: Network Open* 1, no. 5 (September 2018), doi: 0.1001/jamanetworkopen.2018.2327.

13 Xiao-Yang Zhang et al., "Targeting Presynaptic H3 Heteroreceptor in Nucleus Accumbens to Improve Anxiety and Obsessive-Compulsive-Like Behaviors," *Proceedings of the National Academy of Sciences of the United States of America* 117, no. 50 (December 2020): 32155–64, doi: 10.1073/pnas.2008456117.

14 Margaret P. Rayman, "The Importance of Selenium to Human Health," *The Lancet* 356, no. 9225 (July 2000): 233–41, doi: 10.1016/s0140-6736(00)02490-9.

15 Dana Benson, "Thirsty? You're Already Dehydrated," Baylor College of Medicine, June 15, 2015, www.bcm.edu/news/thirsty-you-are-already-dehydrated.

16 L. E. Armstrong et al., "Mild Dehydration Affects Mood in Healthy Young Women," *The Journal of Nutrition* 142, no. 2 (2011): 382–88, doi.org/10.3945/jn.111.142000.

CHAPTER 9: NATURE: LESSONS FROM MOTHER NATURE

1   Margaret Bates, Untitled blog entry, n.d., www.ecopsychology.org/journal/gatherings7/SacredTrees.htm.

2   Suzanne Simard, *Finding the Mother Tree: Discovering the Wisdom of the Forest* (Toronto: Penguin Random House, 2021).

3   Gregory N. Bratman et al., "Nature Experience Reduces Rumination and Subgenual Prefrontal Cortex Activation," *Proceedings of the National Academy of Sciences of the United States of America* 112, no. 28 (July 2015): 8567–72, doi: 10.1073/pnas.1510459112.

4   Danielle F. Shanahan et al., "Health Benefits from Nature Experiences Depend on Dose," *Nature Scientific Reports* 6, no. 28551 (June 2016), doi: 10.1038/srep28551.

5   Genevive R. Meredith et al., "Minimum Time Dose in Nature to Positively Impact the Mental Health of College-Aged Students, and How to Measure It: A Scoping Review," *Frontiers in Psychology* 10 (January 2020), doi:10.3389/fpsyg.2019.02942.

6   Amy L. Sheppard and James S. Wolffsohn, "Digital Eye Strain: Prevalence, Measurement and Amelioration," *British Journal of Ophthalmology* 3, no. 1 (2018): e000146, doi: 10.1136/bmjophth-2018-000146.

7   Virginia E. Sturm et al., "Big Smile, Small Self: Awe Walks Promote Prosocial Positive Emotions in Older Adults," *Emotion* (2020), doi:10.1037/emo0000876.

CHAPTER 10: ONENESS: CONNECTION AND COMPASSION

1   "Loneliness Is a Serious Public-Health Problem," *The Economist*, September 1, 2018, www.economist.com/international/2018/09/01/loneliness-is-a-serious-public -health-problem.

2   G. Oscar Anderson and Colette Thayer, "Loneliness and Social Connections: A National Survey of Adults 45 and Older," AARP Research, American Association of Retired Persons, September 2018, www.aarp.org/research/topics/life/info-2018/loneliness -social-connections.html.

3   Kristina H., "The Vicious Cycle of Loneliness," Medium, March 5, 2019, medium.com/ publishous/the-vicious-cycle-of-loneliness-a9db5b355748.

4   Louise C. Hawkley and John T. Cacioppo, "Loneliness Matters: A Theoretical and Empirical Review of Consequences and Mechanisms," *Annals of Behavioral Medicine* 40, no. 2 (October 2010), doi: 10.1007/s12160-010-9210-8.

5   B. J. Atkinson, "Mindfulness Training and the Cultivation of Secure, Satisfying Couple Relationships," *Couple and Family Psychology: Research and Practice* 2, no. 2 (2013): 73–94, doi: 10.1037/cfp0000002.

6   "Harlow's Classic Studies Revealed the Importance of Maternal Contact," Association for Psychological Science, June 20, 2018, www.psychologicalscience.org/ publications/observer/obsonline/harlows-classic-studies-revealed-the-importance -of-maternal-contact.html. See also Harry F. Harlow, Robert O. Dodsworth, and Margaret K. Harlow, "Total Social Isolation in Monkeys," *Proceedings of the National Academy of Sciences of the United States* 54, no. 1 (1965): 90–97, doi: 10.1073/ pnas.54.1.90.

7   Kathleen C. Lights, Karen M. Grewen, and Janet A. Amico, "More Frequent Partner Hugs and Higher Oxytocin Levels Are Linked to Lower Blood Pressure and Heart Rate in Premenopausal Women," *Biological Psychology* 69, no. 1 (April 2005): 5–21, doi: 10.1016/j.biopsycho.2004.11.002.

8   Ashley E. Thompson, Yvonne Anisimowicz, and Danica Kulibert, "A Kiss Is Worth a Thousand Words: The Development and Validation of a Scale Measuring Motives for Romantic Kissing," *Sexual and Relationship Therapy* 34, no. 1 (August 2019): 54–74, doi:10.1080/14681994.2017.1386299.

9   John Gottman and Nan Silver, *What Makes Love Last?* (New York: Simon & Schuster, 2012).

10 Alison Lynch, "80% of British Women Don't Feel Good Enough, According to New Survey," Metro, August 25, 2015, metro.co.uk/2015/08/25/80-of-british-women- dont-feel-good-enough-according-to-new-survey-5360444/.

11 Tara Brach, *True Refuge: Finding Peace and Freedom in Your Own Awakened Heart* (New York: Bantam, 2013), 163.

12 Paul Bloom, *Against Empathy: The Case for Rational Compassion* (New York: Ecco, 2016).

13 Daniel Goleman and Richard Davidson, *Altered Traits: Science Reveals How Meditation Changes Your Mind, Brain, and Body* (New York: Avery Publishing, 2017).

14 The Karmapa, "The Power of Unbearable Compassion," Lion's Roar, August 23, 2017, www.lionsroar.com/the-power-of-unbearable-compassion/.

15 "Forgiveness: Your Health Depends on It," John Hopkins Medicine, www.hopkinsmedicine.org/health/wellness-and-prevention/forgiveness-your-health-depends-on-it.

16 Loren L. Toussaint, Everett L. Worthington, and David R. Williams, *Forgiveness and Health: Scientific Evidence and Theories Relating Forgiveness to Better Health* (Dordrecht: Springer, 2015).

17 Kathleen A. Lawler-Row et al., "Forgiveness, Physiological Reactivity and Health: The Role of Anger," *International Journal of Psychophysiology* 68, no. 1 (April 2008): 51–58, doi: 10.1016/j.ijpsycho.2008.01.001.

18 Jennifer P. Friedberg, Sonia Suchday, and V. S. Srinivas, "Relationship between Forgiveness and Psychological and Physiological Indices in Cardiac Patients," *International Journal of Behavioral Medicine* 16, no. 3 (February 20, 2009): 205–11, doi: 10.1007/s12529-008-9016-2.

19 Jennifer P. Friedberg, Sonia Suchday, and V. S. Srinivas, "Relationship between Forgiveness and Psychological and Physiological Indices in Cardiac Patients."

20 James W. Carson et al., "Forgiveness and Chronic Low Back Pain: A Preliminary Study Examining the Relationship of Forgiveness to Pain, Anger, and Psychological Distress," *The Journal of Pain* 6, no. 2 (February 2005): 84–91, doi: 10.1016/j.jpain.2004.10.012.

21 Peggy A. Hannon et al., "The Soothing Effects of Forgiveness on Victims' and Perpetrators' Blood Pressure," *Personal Relationships* 19, no. 2 (April 2011): 279–89, doi: 10.1111/j.1475-6811.2011.01356.x.

22 Jennifer P. Friedberg, Sonia Suchday, and V. S. Srinivas, "Relationship between Forgiveness and Psychological and Physiological Indices in Cardiac Patients."

CHAPTER 11: RITUAL AND CREATIVITY: EXPRESSING THE TRUE SELF
1 C. Fogarty and Monisha Vasa, "Restorative Rituals for Mental Health," The Mental Health Collective, March 26, 2019, themhcollective.com/blog/2019/3/26/restorative-rituals-for-mental-health.

2 Meera Bains, "Knitting Takes Off at Addiction Treatment Centre in Surrey as Men Stitch Hundreds of Toques," CBC News, December 22, 2020, www.cbc.ca/news/canada/british-columbia/knitting-takes-off-at-addiction-treatment-centre-in-surrey-as-men-stitch-hundreds-of-toques-1.5851114.

CHAPTER 12: GRATITUDE: EMBRACING THE EVERYDAY
1 C. Nathan DeWall et al., "A Grateful Heart Is a Nonviolent Heart: Cross-Sectional, Experience Sampling, Longitudinal, and Experimental Evidence," *Social Psychological and Personality Science* 3, no. 2 (September 2011): 232–40, doi: 10.1177/1948550611416675.

2 Martin E. P. Seligman et al., "Positive Psychology Progress: Empirical Validation of Interventions," *American Psychologist* 60, no. 5 (July 2005): 410–21, doi: 10.1037/0003-066X.60.5.410.

3 Martin E. P. Seligman et al., "Positive Psychology Progress."

4 Andrea Mathews, "The Closed Mind: Why Does It Close, and How Does It Open?", *Psychology Today* (July 6, 2019), www.psychologytoday.com/ca/blog/traversing-the-inner-terrain/201907/the-closed-mind.

5 Robert A. Emmons and Michael E. McCullough, "Counting Blessings Versus Burdens: An Experimental Investigation of Gratitude and Subjective Well-Being in Daily Life," *Journal of Personality and Social Psychology* 84, no. 2 (February 2003): 377–89, doi: 10.1037//0022-3514.84.2.377.

6　Charles R. Snyder and Shane J. Lopez, *Handbook of Positive Psychology* (Oxford: Oxford University Press, 2011): 848.

7　Alex M. Wood, Jeffrey J. Froh, and Adam W. A. Geraghty, "Gratitude and Well-Being: A Review and Theoretical Integration," *Clinical Psychology Review* 30, no. 7 (November 2010): 890–905, doi: 10.1016/j.cpr.2010.03.005.

8　Alex M. Wood, Jeffrey J. Froh, and Adam W. A. Geraghty, "Gratitude and Well-Being."

9　Susanne Konig and Judith Gluck, "'Gratitude Is with Me All the Time': How Gratitude Relates to Wisdom," *The Journals of Gerontology: Series B* 69, no. 5 (September 2014): 655–66.

10　Melody Beattie, *The Language of Letting Go: Hazelden Meditation Series* (Philadelphia: Hazelden Publishing, 1990).

11　Summer Allen, "The Science of Gratitude," Greater Good Science Center, John Templeton Foundation, May 2018, ggsc.berkeley.edu/images/uploads/GGSC-JTF_White_Paper-Gratitude-FINAL.pdf.

12　Summer Allen, "The Science of Gratitude."

13　Robert A. Emmons and Michael E. McCullough, "Counting Blessings Versus Burdens."

14　Robert A. Emmons and Michael E. McCullough, "Counting Blessings Versus Burdens."

15　Martin E. P. Seligman et al., "Positive Psychology Progress."

16　Martin E. P. Seligman et al., "Positive Psychology Progress."

CHAPTER 13: MAMA SPACE: SELF-REALIZATION AND MOTHERHOOD

1　Dr. Shefali, *The Conscious Parent: Transforming Ourselves, Empowering Our Children* (Vancouver: Namaste Publishing, 2010).

2　"Postpartum Depression," Anxiety & Depression Association of America, adaa.org/living-with-anxiety/women/postpartum-depression.

3　Marion Righetti-Veltema et al., "Postpartum Depression and Mother-Infant Relationship at 3 Months Old," *Journal of Affective Disorders* 70, no. 3 (August 2002): 291–306, doi: www.sciencedirect.com/science/article/abs/pii/S0165032701003676.

4　G. Stern and L. Kruckman, "Multi-Disciplinary Perspective on Post-Partum Depression: An Anthropological Critique," *Social Science Medicine* 17, no. 15 (1983): 1027–41, doi: 10.1016/0277-9536(83)90408-2.

5　Marion Righetti-Veltema et al., "Postpartum Depression and Mother-Infant Relationship at 3 Months Old."

Index

role in, 57; power of, 184–86; sound and, 111–12; strengthening, 186–89; top takeaways about, 201. *See also* relationships

conscious motherhood, 234–35

consciousness, 73, 88, 96, 108–11, 233–34

Conscious Parent, The (Shefali), 234–35

contemplative meditation, 54–55

control, 80–81

Cornell University, 175

cortisol: alcohol increases, 157; breath work reduces, 101; dangers of, 21, 22; dehydration increases, 165; in fight-or-flight response, 23; function, 20–21; influence on brain plasticity, 83; kissing reduces, 189. *See also* fight-or-flight response

COVID-19 pandemic, 44, 184, 231–33

cravings, food, 157, 159–60

creativity, 206–12; journaling about, 213; Karyn's story, 203–5, 212; meditation and, 58, 210–12; Michele's experience with, 208; power of, 206–9; Shona's story, 216; top takeaways about, 213

criticism. *See* self-criticism

cruciferous vegetables, 156

cuddle neurochemical, 20, 131, 188

culture. *See* Western culture

Dalai Lama, 120

danger. *See* fight-or-flight response

darkness, 128–29, 136

dark night, 42

Davis, Angela, 15

deer, 177

dehydration, 165

depression, 57, 220, 240–41

design, 174–75

detachment. *See* equanimity

determined practice, 116

dharma names, 81

dieting, 154. *See also* food

discrimination, 121

distraction, 62. *See also* patterns of thinking and feeling

dopamine, 19, 130, 188–89, 219

dreams, 28–29, 77, 208, 216

dream yoga, 138–39

dukkha. See suffering

Eastern spiritual traditions, 56. *See also* Buddhism

eating. *See* food

Economist, 184

ecotherapy, 175

egoic mind: food and, 157; meditation and, 61, 67; mindfulness and, 73, 74; self-criticism of, 61, 173, 190, 209; self-limitations of, 207

8 sacred soul qualities, 221–23, 228–30

Eightfold Path, 81

Emma (client), 231–33, 242–43

Emmons, Robert A., 220, 223–24

emotional intelligence, 57

emotions: equanimity and dealing with, 85–86; fear, 62, 73, 185, 220; guilt, 7; gut health and, 154–55; happiness, 75–76, 154; invoked by words, 111–12; primary, 218; Sudarshan Kriya and positive, 102. *See also* anger; love; patterns of thinking and feeling

empathy, 191

encouragement. *See* notes of encouragement

endorphins, 19, 95, 129

energy, 157, 158

epinephrine. *See* adrenaline

equanimity, 84–88; defined, 84; food and, 157; journaling about, 88, 89; Kendra's story, 88; meditation and, 62, 66, 86–88; mind chatter and, 84–85, 88; progressive muscle relaxation and, 45; sleep and, 131–32; top takeaways about, 89

essential oils, 45, 131

European Union, 15

eustress, 21–22

exercise, 129

exercises, 7. *See also* breathing exercises; invitations to practice; mantras; meditation exercises; relaxation techniques

expansion mantras, 118

expectations, 59

Fabergé Organics commercial, 247

families. *See* motherhood; relationships

father/daughter relationships, 34, 72

fatigue, 57, 124

fear, 62, 73, 185, 220

feet, 38–39

feminism and stress, 13–16
fertility issues, 232, 239–40
fiber-rich foods, 156, 159, 160
Fight Club (Palahniuk), 123
fight-or-flight response: amygdala's role in, 22–23; breath and, 95, 98, 101; cold extremities, 38; dehydration activates, 165; positive stress and, 21; purpose, 17; Vooo chanting and, 18. *See also* adrenaline; cortisol
Finding Inner Calm through Water (meditation exercise), 166–67
Finding True Self in Nature (meditation exercise), 178–80
food, 147–68; affection *vs.*, 188; approach to, 149–50, 154; gut health and, 154–56, 158, 160; as healing, 153–54; journaling about, 153, 159, 168; Lara's story, 147–49, 168; meditation exercises for, 151–52, 166–67; mindfulness and, 153, 157, 163–64; nutrients for nervous system health, 160–63; sleep and, 129, 134, 136–37, 143–44; stimulants, 129, 143–44, 149, 156, 157–60, 161; top takeaways about, 168; water's role in quenching anxiety, 164–66
forest bathing, 176–77
forgiveness. *See* self-forgiveness
Framingham Study, 96
Frontiers of Psychology, 57
fructose, 159
fruits, 136, 137, 156, 159
future events. *See* patterns of thinking and feeling

gamma-aminobutyric acid (GABA), 19, 134–35
Gandhi, Indira, 51
gender differences, 14, 35, 132
gender inequality. *See* patriarchy and gender inequality
golden turmeric latte, 129
Goleman, Daniel, 191
Gottman, John, 189
governments, 15
gratitude, 215–30; brain and, 219–20; journaling about, 219–20, 223–24, 228–30; meditation exercise for, 225–27; Michele's experience with, 240; power of, 217–18; role in relationships, 186; sacred soul qualities of, 221–23,

228–30; Shona's story, 215–17, 227; top takeaways about, 228; wisdom and, 218
growth. *See* self-realization
guilt, 7
gut health, 154–56, 158, 160

hands, 38–39
Hanh, Thich Nhat, 91
happiness, 75–76, 154
happiness neurochemical. *See* serotonin
Harlow, Harry, 188
Hawaii, 196
healing, 33–50; autogenic training, 39–42; breathing exercise for, 37–38; through conscious breath, 93–94; food's role in, 153–54; journaling about, 50; masculine *vs.* feminine, 35; Michele's story, 33–34, 49; overview of biofeedback, 35–36; progressive muscle relaxation, 44–49; self-realization stages, 42–43; through sound, 112–13 (*see also* mantras); top takeaways about, 49
healing mantras, 118
Healing Power of Gratitude, The (meditation exercise), 225–27
healthism, 16
heart attacks, 196
heart disease, 57
HeartMath, 36
heart rate, 95, 129
heart rhythm, 36
Hermit, The (book), 6
higher purpose, 43
honesty, 30, 68, 84, 189
Ho'oponopono (meditation exercise), 196–201
hormones. *See* melatonin; neurochemicals
Horne, Jim, 132
hugging, 188
Human Performance Laboratory, 165

ignorance, 218
Illuminating as Light (meditation exercise), 210–12
imagery exercises, 7. *See also* meditation exercises; relaxation techniques
impermanence, 219
inception, 42
injuries, 34, 49, 123–24

inner critics. *See* self-criticism
insomnia, 123
integration, 43
intentions: concluding, 252; in
meditation, 59-60; as reference
points, 3; in ritual, 205, 206; sleep
and, 130, 138
internal abundance, 221-22, 229
intersection of oppression, 15
invitations to practice: approach
to, 5-6; calling in sacred ritual,
206; mantras, 119-20; mastering
posture, 59; mindful eating, 163-64;
strengthening connection, 187-89;
tracking stimulants, 159-60; Vooo
chanting, 18. *See also* breathing
exercises; meditation exercises;
relaxation techniques
iodine, 163

Jacobson, Edmund, 44
Japanese wisdom, 176
Jen (client), 51-53, 68
jet lag, 127, 136
Jewel in the Lotus, The (mantra), 120
Johns Hopkins University, 54
Jones, Claudia, 15
journaling: approach to, 5; boundaries
surrounding, 235; breath, 105;
connection, 202; creativity, 213;
dreams, 29, 139; equanimity, 88,
89; food, 153, 159, 168; gratitude,
219-20, 223-24, 228-30; healing, 50;
meditation, 60, 69; mindfulness, 89;
motherhood, 243; nature, 181; ritual,
213; self-forgiveness, 202; sleep, 145;
sound, 112, 122; stress, 31; worries,
130
Journal of Attention Disorders, 57
judgment. *See* patterns of thinking
and feeling; self-criticism
Jung, Carl, 184

Karmapa, Seventeenth, 192
Karma Rigzen Lhamo, 81
Karyn (client), 203-5, 212
kefir, 156
Kendra (client), 71-72, 88
Killingsworth, Matt, 76
kimchi, 156
kissing, 188-89
kiwis, 136

knitting, 207
kombucha, 156

lamas, 6, 120
Lara (client), 147-49, 168
lavender essential oil, 45, 131
Levine, Peter, 18, 124
LGBTQIA+ people, 148, 185
light, 127-29, 132, 137, 175, 210-12
limbic system: amygdala, 17, 22, 83, 160;
function, 17; sleep and, 130, 131
Lloyd (therapy dog), 108, 172-73
locus of control, 80-81
loneliness, 184-85
Lori (client), 91-93, 104
lotus, 216-17, 227
love, 186, 187, 191, 195, 196-201
Love and Radiance Meditation
(meditation exercise), 249-51
loving-kindness meditation, 55, 67,
236-38
lucid dreaming, 138
lung capacity, 96, 101

magnesium, 135, 161
Mahayana Buddhism, 216
maitri (loving kindness), 55-56
mantras, 113-20; closed-eye mantra
meditation, 119; cultivating a practice
of, 115-16; defined, 114; emotions
invoked by, 111; examples, 117-18;
in Ho'oponopono, 196-201; for
motherhood, 238-39; Om Mani Padme
Hum, 120; Premal on, 107; at Ram
Dass's retreat, 113-14; for ritual, 206;
for sleep, 131; top takeaways about,
121. *See also* sound
marriage, 14. *See also* relationships
Mason, Konda, 8
Maya (client), 11-13, 30
meal plans, 153-54
meditation, 51-69; approach to, 56;
becoming wholeheartedly ourselves,
53-55; benefits, 54-55, 56-58;
boundaries surrounding, 235;
cultivating a practice of, 3-4, 59-62; in
healing trauma, 6, 66; Jen's story, 51-53,
68; journaling about, 60, 69; Metta,
55, 67; retreats for, 67-68, 177; role in
relationships, 186-87; Shona's story,
216; sleep and, 62, 138-43; Tonglen, 67,
192-95; top takeaways about, 68

meditation exercises: Anapanasati, 63–66; Arriving into Present Time, 78–79; The Artemis Within, 171–72; Awakening Our Dreams, 28–29; closed-eye mantra meditation, 119; Finding Inner Calm through Water, 166–67; Finding True Self in Nature, 178–80; The Healing Power of Gratitude, 225–27; Ho'oponopono, 196–201; Illuminating as Light, 210–12; Love and Radiance Meditation, 249–51; Metta for Mothers, 236–38; Rewriting Your Food Story, 151–52; The River of Awareness, 26–27; Sound Consciousness, 110–11; Tonglen Meditation, 193–95; Training the Mind for Equanimity, 86–88; Vipassana, 139–43; walking meditation, 174; The Welcoming, 8–9

melatonin: bedroom temperature and, 130; food sources of, 136–37, 162; light and, 127–28, 129, 132; supplements for, 135–36

memory, 57, 73

mental health, approach to, 1–9

Metta for Mothers (meditation exercise), 236–38

Metta meditation, 55, 67

milk, 137

mind-body system, approach to, 2, 5, 16

mind chatter and wandering. See patterns of thinking and feeling

mindfulness, 71–84; to counter self-criticism, 173; food and, 153, 157, 163–64; gratitude and, 220, 221, 229; journaling about, 89; Kendra's story, 71–72; living in the present, 73–77; locus of control and, 80–81; meditation exercise for, 78–79; nature and, 177; note of encouragement on, 58; and reshaping the brain, 82–84; ripple effect, 81–82; ritual and, 205–6; role in relationships, 186, 187; sound and, 109, 121; top takeaways about, 89

mirroring, 124

miscarriages, 239–40

Modernist architecture, 175

monkeys, 188

mood, 57, 74–76

morning larks, 127

morning mantras, 117

motherhood, 231–43; approach to, 233; conscious, 234–35; Emma's story, 231–33, 242–43; Harlow's monkey study and, 188; journaling about, 243; loss of children, 215–16, 227, 239–40; mantras for, 238–39; Maya's story, 12; meditation exercise for, 236–38; Michele's story, 239–40; postpartum mental health issues, 240–42; top takeaways about, 243; work and, 92, 124, 231–33, 243

mouth breathing, 98

muscles, 44–49

musical instruments, 113

Nadi Shodhana (breathing exercise), 98–100

narratives. See patterns of thinking and feeling; self-criticism

National Institute of Mental Health, 14

nature, 169–81; Artemis's story, 169–70, 180; design and, 174–75; forest bathing, 176–77; getting back to, 172–74; journaling about, 181; meditation exercises for, 171–72, 174, 178–80; top takeaways about, 180

Nature Scientific Reports, 175

nervous system: GABA and, 134; gut and, 154; nutrients for, 160–63; overview of central, 16–18; sleep and, 125, 129, 131. See also parasympathetic nervous system; sympathetic nervous system

neurochemicals: acetylcholine, 18; dopamine, 19, 130, 188–89, 219; endorphins, 19, 95, 219; GABA, 19, 134–35; norepinephrine, 189; overview of, 19–21; oxytocin, 20, 131, 188. See also adrenaline; cortisol; serotonin

neuroplasticity, 82–84, 191

New York University, 85

night owls, 127

norepinephrine, 189

nose breathing, 95, 98

notes of encouragement: boundaries, 235; breath work, 104; countering self-criticism, 173; determined practice, 116; food, 153; impermanence, 219; inner wisdom, 209; mindfulness, 58; self-care, 7, 82; self-realization, 42–43, 248;

34, 72, 217. *See also* connection; motherhood; self-relationships

relaxation techniques: autogenic training, 39-42; as biofeedback method, 36; patriarchal, 35; progressive muscle relaxation, 44-49

Remen, Rachel Naomi, 33

resilience: anxiety's role in, 24; brain plasticity's role in, 83; gratitude and, 217, 218; Shona's story, 216; Shu's story, 144

resistance, 4, 5, 42, 52.

See also self-criticism

respiratory health, 96

rest-and-repair response, 17, 18

restless legs syndrome, 135

retreats, 33, 34, 67-68, 113-14, 177

Return to Calm (relaxation technique), 40-42

Rewriting Your Food Story (meditation exercise), 151-52

ripple effect, 81-82

rising. *See* self-realization

ritual: bedtime, 128-33; gratitude as, 223, 229; journaling about, 213; Karyn's story, 212; mindfulness and, 205-6; top takeaways about, 213

River of Awareness, The (meditation exercise), 26-27

Rubin Museum of Art, 109

rumination. *See* patterns of thinking and feeling

sacred soul qualities, 221-23, 228-30

safety, 17

Salima (client), 107-8, 121

Salzberg, Sharon, 11

sanctuaries, 196

San Diego State University, 80

sand tray therapy, 184, 201

sankhara (conditions of the mind), 66. *See also* patterns of thinking and feeling

sauerkraut, 156

Schultz, Johannes Heinrich, 39-40

seeds, 137

selenium, 163

self-acceptance, 104, 190-91

self-care: desire for, 82, 150; guilt surrounding, 7

self-compassion: to counter self-criticism, 173; Jen's story, 52;

loneliness and, 185; mindful eating as, 164; self-acceptance, 190-91; and shift in female consciousness, 233

self-criticism: countering, 173, 217-18; Maya's story, 12; meditation and, 55, 60, 61; Michele's experience with, 33; narratives of "lack," 190, 209, 239; on sleep, 132. *See also* patterns of thinking and feeling

self-forgiveness, 195-201; benefits, 195-96; journaling about, 202; meditation exercise for, 196-201; top takeaways about, 202

self-gratitude, 217

self-honesty, 30, 68, 84, 189

self-knowledge. *See* awareness; wisdom

self-limitations, 207

self-love, 195, 196-201

self-realization, 245-52; approach to, 1-9; "Buddha" means, 125; concluding intention, 252; description of, 246-47; importance of using your voice, 247-48; meditation exercise for, 249-51; stages, 42-43

self-regulation, 36

self-relationships: Lori's story, 92; meditation and, 53, 68; Michele's story, 34; nature of, 24, 25

self-soothing, 94, 131-32

self-worth, 92-93, 104, 190, 195, 221

Seligman, Martin, 224

serotonin: alcohol reduces, 157; food sources of, 137, 162; function, 20; gratitude increases, 219; gut's role in producing, 154

sex, 58

sexism, 15. *See also* patriarchy and gender inequality

sexual harassment, 15

shampoo commercial, 247

Shari (wisdom teacher), 99

shecession, 232

Shefali, Dr., 231, 234-35

shinrin-yoku (forest bathing), 176-77

Shona (client), 215-17, 227

short-term stress, 21-22

Shu (client), 123-24, 143-44

Siddhartha, 153. *See also* Buddha

silent retreats, 67-68

Simard, Suzanne, 174

sitting, 59

Situ Rinpoche, Tai, 81-82

6-second kiss, 188–89

sleep, 123–45; boundaries surrounding, 235; chronotypes, 126–27, 133; dream yoga, 138–39; forgiveness and, 196; journaling about, 145; meditation and, 62, 138–43; Michele's experience with, 208; nutrients for, 134–37; physiology of, 125–27; Shu's story, 123–24, 143–44; sleep deprivation, 123–24, 126, 128, 143; sleep hygiene, 128–33; sleep-wake cycle, 127, 133, 136; top takeaways about, 144

Sleepfaring (Horne), 132

Sleep Foundation, 132

social jet lag, 127

somatic psychotherapy, 44

somatic therapy, 216

songs. *See* mantras

sound, 107–13; connection and, 111–12; healing through, 112–13; journaling about, 112, 122; as part of human consciousness, 108–9; Salima's story, 107–8, 121; sound baths, 112; top takeaways about, 121; Vooo chanting, 18. *See also* mantras

Sound Consciousness (meditation exercise), 110–11

soybeans, 156

soy milk, 137

spiritual health, approach to, 1–9

"Stillness" (poem), 245

stimulants. *See* food: stimulants

stories. *See* patterns of thinking and feeling; self-criticism

stress, 11–31; auditory system and, 107–8; becomes anxiety, 22–25; brain plasticity and, 83; as feminist issue, 13–16; forgiveness and, 196; gratitude and, 218, 220; gut health and, 155; journaling about, 31; magnesium levels and, 161; Maya's story, 11–13, 30; meditation exercises for, 26–29; overview of central nervous system and, 16–18; overview of neurochemicals and, 19–21; patriarchal methods of reducing, 35; positive *vs.* negative, 21–22; sleep and, 132–33; subjectivity of, 35–36; top takeaways about, 30

stress hormones. *See* adrenaline; cortisol

stroke, 57

structuring practices, 23

Sudarshan Kriya (breathing exercise), 101–3

suffering: in Buddhism, 25, 84; desire to free others from, 191, 222, 229; meditation exercises for relieving, 193–95; primary emotions driving, 218. *See also* pain and trauma

sugar, 149, 156, 158–59

Sujata (woman who fed Siddhartha), 153

superfoods, 155–56

supplements, 134, 135–36, 161

support systems, 241–42

survival hormone. *See* adrenaline

sustenance. *See* food

symbols, 216–17, 227

sympathetic nervous system, 17, 18, 93, 155. *See also* fight-or-flight response

Tai Situ Rinpoche, 81–82

taking refuge, 81

tea, 129, 134, 144, 156

technology, 74–76, 129–30, 143–44, 176

temperature, 130

therapy dogs, 108, 172–73

Thoreau, Henry David, 29, 169

thoughts. *See* patterns of thinking and feeling

Tibetan Buddhism, 81

Tibetan instruments, 113

Tolle, Eckhart, 71

Tonglen meditation, 67, 192–95

toques, 207

Training the Mind for Equanimity (meditation exercise), 86–88

transformation. *See* self-realization

trauma. *See* pain and trauma

trees, 174

true self: nature and, 172, 178–80; nature of, 73, 88; self-compassion and, 190; as stage in self-realization, 43. *See also* creativity; ritual

tryptophan, 137, 162

turmeric, 129

Twenge, Jean, 80

20-second habits, 187–89

Ujjayi Pranayama (breathing exercise), 37–38

United States, 14, 175, 177, 184–85, 196

University of California, 113

University of Connecticut, 165

vagus nerve, 17–18, 93–94, 99, 155
validation, 12, 80–81
vegetables, 156, 159
vibrational sound, 111–12, 113
violence, 14, 204, 212
Vipassana (meditation exercise), 139–43
vitamin B6, 136
vitamin D, 128, 137, 161
voice, 30, 121, 148, 243, 247–48. *See also* creativity
Vooo chanting, 18
vulnerability, 189

Walden (Thoreau), 169
walking meditation, 174
Washington state, 177
water, 132, 135, 164–67
weighted blankets, 130–31
Welcoming, The (meditation exercise), 8–9
Western culture: approach to, 2, 3; approach to meditation, 56; breath undervalued in, 95; diet, 153–54, 157, 161; gratitude and, 223, 224; lack of support for new moms in, 242; sleep in, 125, 127; social expectations of women in, 15–16; trends in locus of control, 80–81; women's stress levels in, 13–14
Wigmore, Ann, 147
wildness. *See* nature
Willis-Ekbom disease, 135
wisdom: of adversity, 223, 229; bodily, 165; in breath work, 102; gratitude and, 218; inner, 6–7, 209; meditation's role in, 54; nature and, 169–70, 174, 176, 177, 180. *See also* awareness
wisdom mantras, 117
women: approach to health of, 1–9; society's expectations of, 13, 15–16; stress as feminist issue, 13–16; struggles faced by, 6–7, 13–15, 25, 232
Women, Race & Class (Davis), 15
words and sound, 111–12
work: gender differences in, 14; motherhood and, 92, 124, 231–33, 243; sexual harassment at, 15
working memory, 57
World Is Sound, The (art exhibition), 109
worry journal, 130

worthiness. *See* self-worth
writing. *See* journaling

Yale University, 191
yoga: breath and, 37, 96; dream yoga, 138–39; retreats for, 33, 34; sound healing in, 112
yogic science, 101
You Must Relax (Jacobson), 44

Zazen Counting Breath (breathing exercise), 97
Zen Buddhism, 91, 97

ABOUT THE AUTHOR

DR. MICHELE KAMBOLIS is an acclaimed author and speaker who has been featured on *Good Morning America*, Huff Post Live, Goop, and Raw Beauty Talks. She holds a PhD in mind-body medicine. She has been a clinical counselor for more than twenty years, and her evidence-based resources will set you on a path of self-healing, inner wisdom, and profound mind-body health. Her first book, *Generation Stressed: Play-Based Tools to Help Your Child Overcome Anxiety*, was widely praised by readers and critics alike. She lives and works in Vancouver, Canada.